Sacred Sound Formulas

TO AWAKEN THE MODERN MIND

SANSKRIT MANTRA TECHNIQUES
TO RAISE YOUR VIBRATION

PARASHAKTI JILL JARDINE
WITH DR. ALEXI JARDINE MARTEL

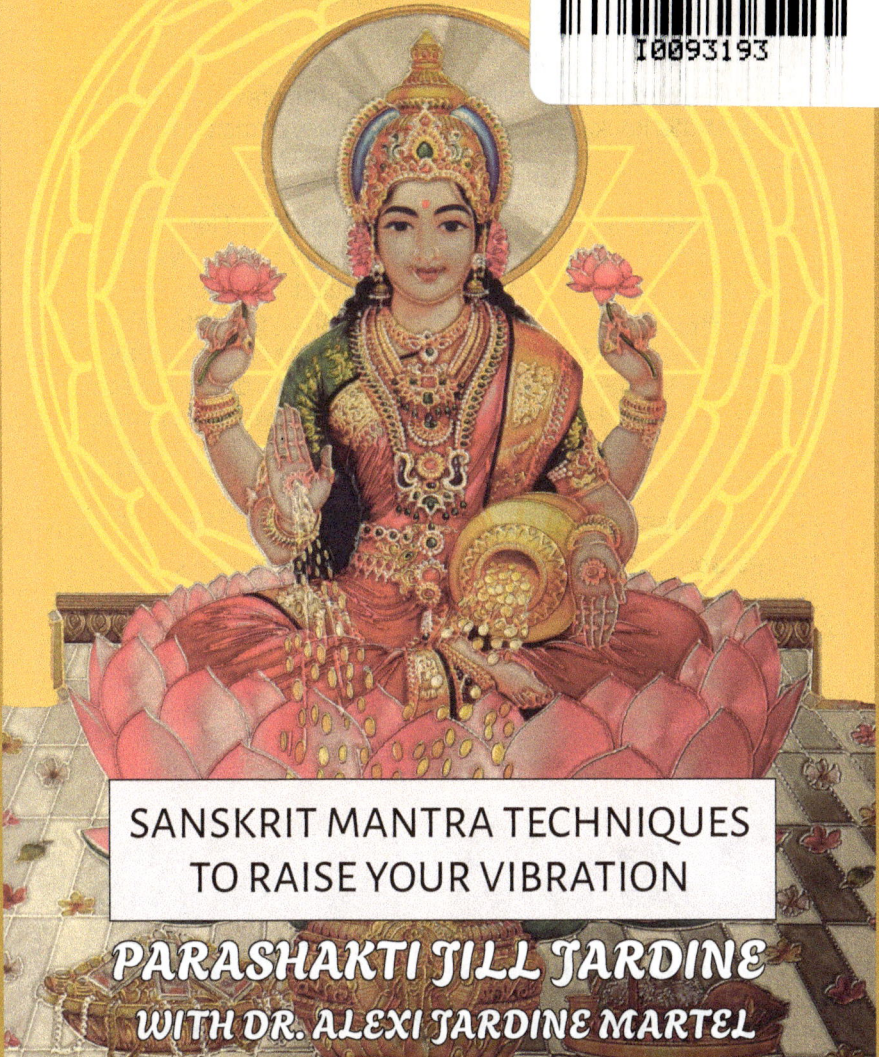

ISBN: 978-1-958150-51-1
Sacred Sound Formulas to Awaken the Modern Mind: Sanskrit Mantra Techniques to Raise your Vibration

October 2025

Published by Inner Peace Press
Eau Claire, Wisconsin, USA
www.innerpeacepress.com

This book is dedicated to Mother:

Divine Mother,

my spiritual Mother, Guru Rama Mata,

and my first guru, Elsa Jardine

reader reviews

"I am delighted that Namadeva's student, Parashakti Jill, has written this comprehensive book of mantras. It carries forward the lineage brought to the West by my husband, Sadguru Sant Keshavadas, and transmitted to Namadeva. With devotion and clarity, this book makes the sacred mantras accessible to all, honoring their ancient roots while offering practical guidance for modern seekers. I am grateful to see this lineage carried forward with such devotion and care."

GURU RAMA MATA
Vishwa Shanti Ashram, Bangalore, India

"As an intuitive astrologer and psychic with 30+ years as an internationally respected counselor, Jill Jardine's *Sacred Sound Formulas to Awaken the Modern Mind* provides excellent instructions on the use of Sanskrit mantra as simple yet powerful tools to help resolve a wide range of practical and spiritual challenges. Building upon the teachings of the lineage of Sadguru Sant Keshavadas and Namadeva Acharya, these teachings can enable self-empowerment that aids with many life challenges."

BHARATA BILL FRANCIS BARRY
Vedic Priest & Spiritual Counselor, Pujari, and Mantra Teacher in Namadeva's lineage

"I was introduced to Sanskrit mantras by Jill Jardine in 2008, and later studied with her teacher, Namadeva Acharya. The first chant I learned, Aham Prema – the mantra for love – changed my life. After just two days of chanting, I met my boyfriend, proof of how powerful these practices can be. Mantras became so essential that I included one at the beginning of every chapter of my book, *Shot@Love: A Celebrity Photographer's Unfiltered Lens on Dating and Finding Love*. Jill's teachings appear throughout, and she has been a recurring guest on my Shot At Love podcast, where her wisdom continues to inspire listeners worldwide. Jill's devotion to this sacred lineage has changed me profoundly, and I know this book will help others find love and create deeper fulfillment in their own journeys."

KERRY BRETT

Award-Winning Photographer, Podcaster, and Best-Selling Author

"Namadeva's teachings through Jill have been a guiding light on my spiritual journey for many years. Jill has shared powerful transmissions and wisdom, and guided me to my Vedic Astrology gurus Komilla Sutton and Dr. Gary Gomes. Jill's expertise and insight in Sanskrit mantra teachings and astrology are truly invaluable resources."

EDWIN VEGUILLA

Vedic Astrologer

Contents

lineage

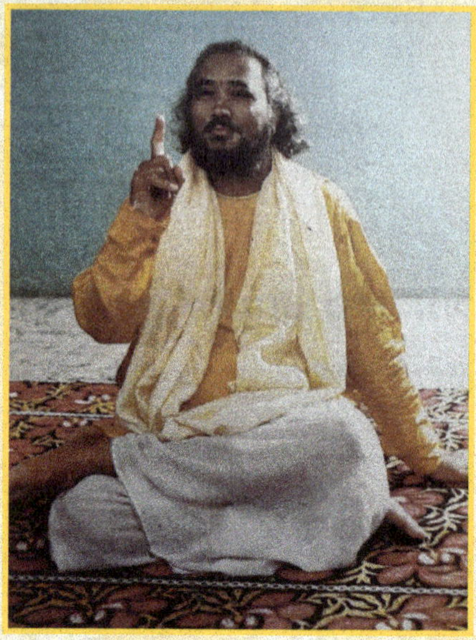

SADGURU SANT KESHAVADAS
Founder of the Temple of Cosmic religion, belonged to the ancient line of singing saints and exemplifies the tradition of Bhakti Yoga, or devotional mysticism. Author of more than 45 books and composer of over 45,000 spiritual songs in Sanskrit and other languages. Mantra Guru to Namadeva Acharya, husband of Guru Rama Mata, and father of Sri Muralidhar Pai.

NAMADEVA ACHARYA, THOMAS ASHLEY-FARRAND
One of the Western world's foremost authorities on the application of Sanskrit mantra to life's problems. Namadeva authored many books and audio programs including *Healing Mantras*, *Shakti Mantras*, and *Chakra Mantras*.

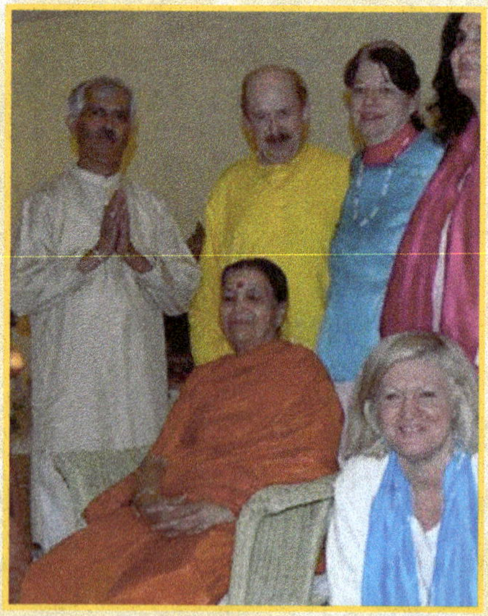

GURU GATHERING OF MANTRA LINEAGE IN BOSTON IN 2010: (Standing from left to right: Sri Muralidhar Pai, Namadeva Acharya, Satyabhama, Shivani Silvia Sune; Seated: Guru Rama Mata, Parashakti Jill Jardine)

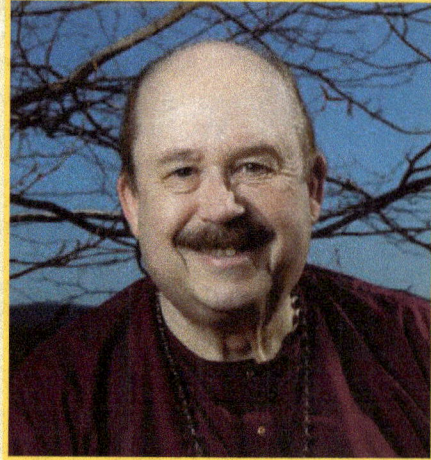

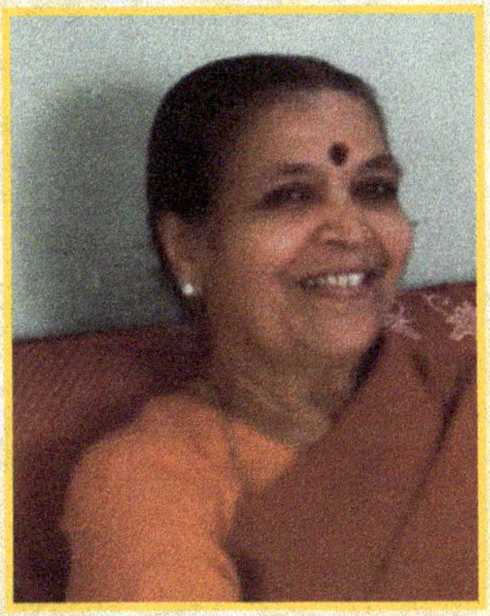

GURU RAMA MATA
Gurumataji Rama Mata became the successor to Sant Keshavadas after his Maha Samadhi in 1997. She is the President of the Temple of Cosmic Religion and continues to administer its world headquarters at Vishwa Shanti Ashram in Bangalore, India.

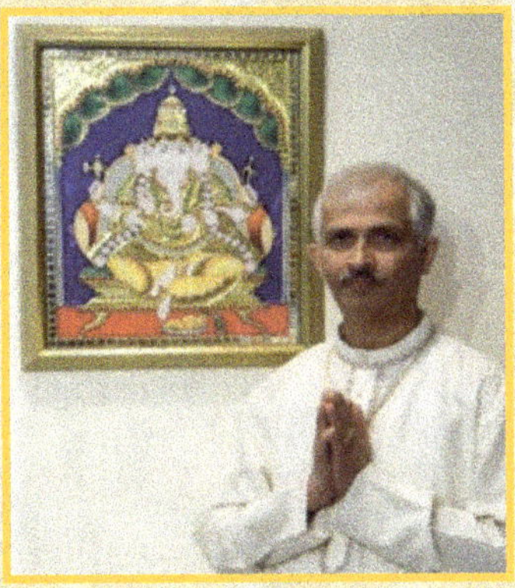

SRI MURALIDHAR PAI
Murali is a Vedic Priest, Pujari, and mantra teacher. He is one of the most accomplished Indian classical musicians in the U.S. and has performed with celebrities in the world of Indian classical music. A guru in his own right, Murali continues the teachings of the lineage, while sharing his powerful Mantra and Tabla Shakti.

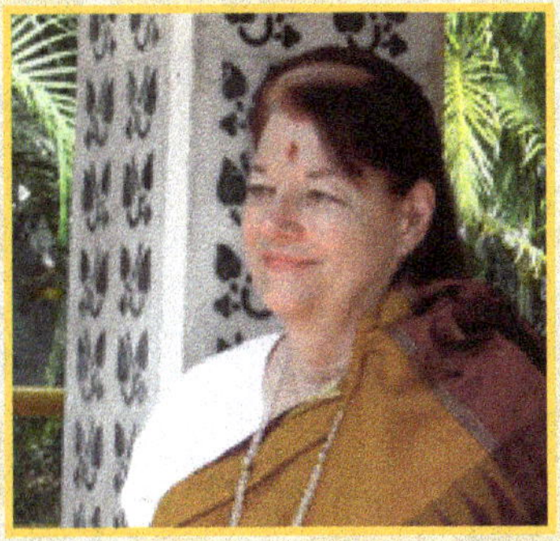

SATYABHAMA ASHLEY-FARRAND
Wife of Thomas Ashley-Farrand and founder of Saraswati Publications which distributed his teachings. Pujari and Priest of Gayatri Temple in Albuquerque, NM, until her passing in 2025.

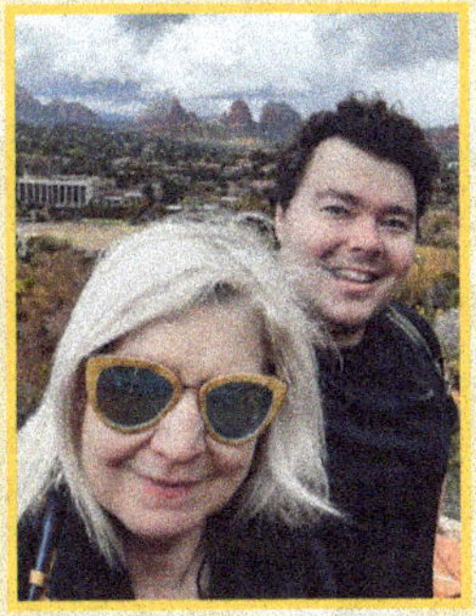

DR. ALEXI JARDINE MARTEL (with Parashakti Jill Jardine) Professor of Psychology. Dr. Martel is a second generation certified Sanskrit Mantra instructor through the lineage of Sanatana Dharma Satsang and a Professional Vedic Astrologer.

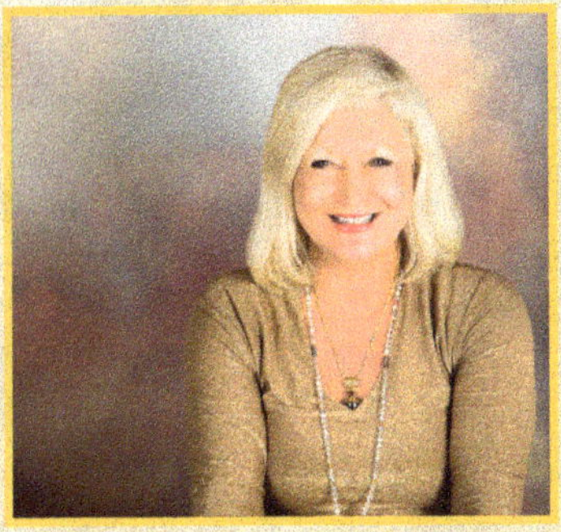

REVEREND PARASHAKTI JILL JARDINE
Student and devotee of Namadeva Acharya, Guru Rama Mata, and Sri Muralidhar Pai. Sponsor of their workshops in the Boston area. Yoga teacher. Certified Sanskrit Mantra instructor through Sanatana Dharma Satsang.

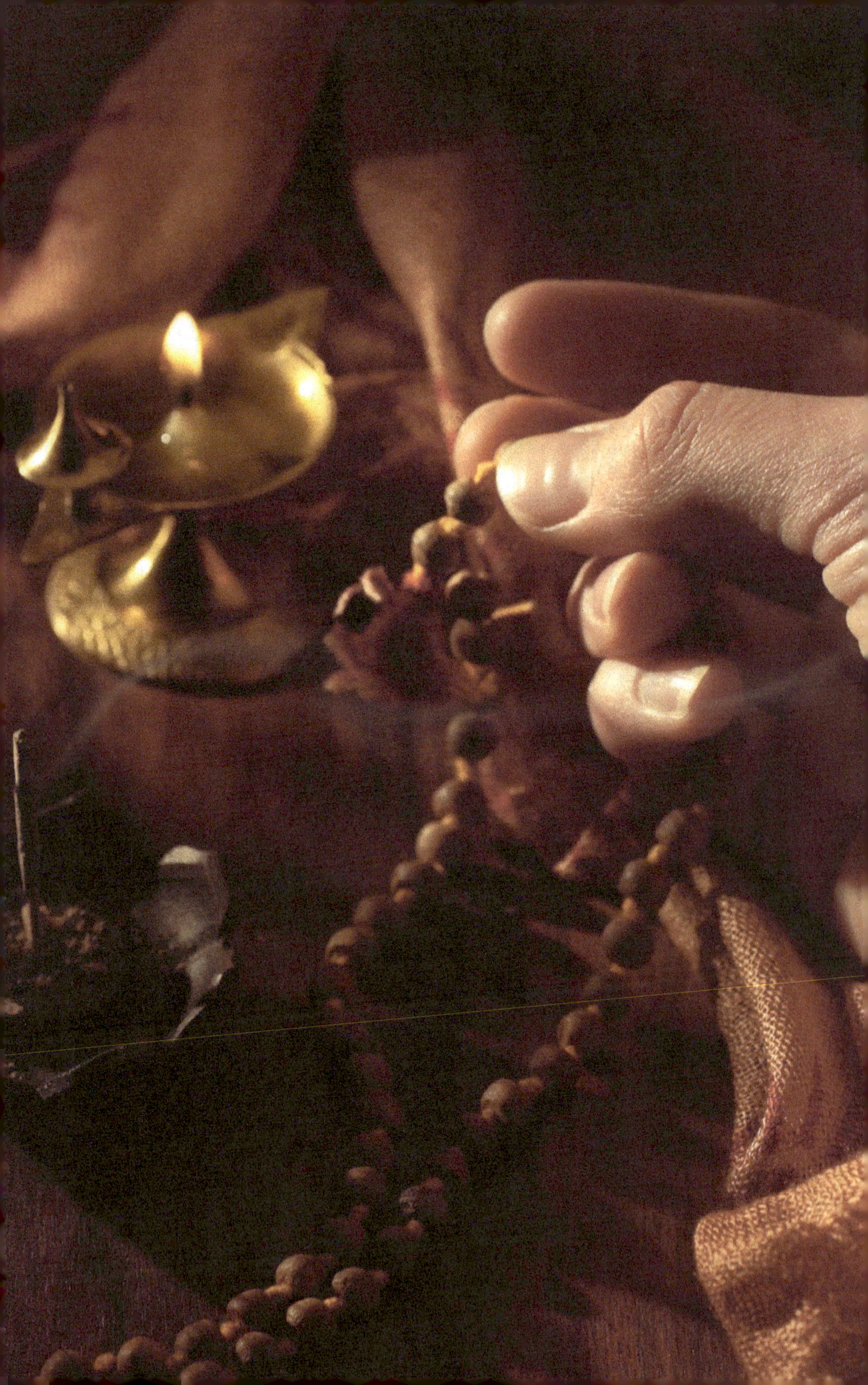

introduction

This book offers profound techniques that will help you shift your frequency to align with the higher vision for your life. It is being written now because it is the time on the planet when we need it. Years ago I was told by my **mantra** teacher, Thomas-Ashley Farrand, Namadeva Acharya, known simply as Namadeva by his students, that there would come a time when chanting mantras would be embraced and effective in restoring righteous universal order (also known as **world dharma**) on planet Earth. That time is now.

The ancient healing transmission of **Sanskrit** mantras and their encoded power can help restore personal as well as planetary well-being. I am honored to offer this time-tested technique through words and chants. Sanskrit mantra chanting is the oldest existing form of chanting for which we have records. Sanskrit mantras existed prior to the development of writing. Chanting Sanskrit mantras can raise your vibration and clear subconscious blocks which interfere with aspirations and goals.

As Namadeva wrote, "mantras are powerful, they are formidable, they work." This has been my experience after years of chanting Sanskrit mantras as passed down from my lineage of Sanskrit mantra gurus. I have been initiated through these mantra gurus who transmitted these sacred

definitions of **bold words** can be found in the glossary at end of book sound formulas. It is my honor and personal **dharma** (one's soul's mission on Earth in alignment with universal righteous order) to share them with you now.

In order to receive the full benefit of Sanskrit mantras, one must learn them or listen to them transmitted by a qualified teacher or guru, one who has been initiated in this ancient yogic path by a true guru or teacher of mantra. This is because there is a special transmission of energy, called **shakti**, divine life force, which flows from the teacher while chanting to the recipient or student of the mantra.

I am a certified Sanskrit mantra instructor through the lineage of Namadeva Acharya, and his teachers Sadguru Sant Keshavadas and Guru Rama Mata, and their son, Sri Muralidhar Pai. And have the esteemed privilege of being given their *darshan*. A chapter later in this book features Muralidhar Pai, or Muraliji for his devotees, and expands on the gurus of this mantra lineage.

I am guided to fill the void with books on mantras in Namadeva's tradition. I come at this from my work as a professional counseling astrologer and therapist who has shared these mantras as remedial measures for thousands of clients and students over the years. I am humbled by the body of work Namadeva passed down to us, picking up where his teacher Sadguru Sant Keshavadas left off, who predeceased him and released an incredible compendium on mantras and teachings of this lineage: Sanatana Dharma Satsang through Vishwa Shanti Ashram.

As the humble student of Namadeva Acharya, I will do my best to transmit his teachings. Namadeva left his body in 2010, and his final published book on Sanskrit mantras was written in 2006. I have felt the void of there being no more books of his to read, after reading his books over and over again, and sharing them with many people. Namadeva's influential titles are: *Healing Mantras* (1999), *Shakti Mantras* (2003), *Chakra Mantras* (2006), and *Mantra Meditation: Change Your Karma with the Power of Sacred Sound* (2006).

What I have learned and experienced is: Mantras Rock! They offer so many benefits including peace of mind, release of anxieties, emotional and mental healing, physical health and well-being, enhanced life force, better relationships, and increased prosperity – concepts I share in this book.

Mantras were originally composed in Sanskrit. While this book does not include the original script, it provides transliterations and pronunciation guides to help you accurately vocalize the mantras. Sanskrit itself is a powerful tool for engaging with the subtle energy body.

This book carries forth the living tradition of Sanskrit mantra, as it was reverently transmitted to me by Namadeva who continued the sacred work of his mantra guru, Sadguru Sant Keshavadas. However, this book differs from those of my predecessors in that it draws upon my experience as an astrologer, counselor, and therapist, having prescribed thousands of Sanskrit mantras to clients seeking to take an active role in their healing and the expansion of their consciousness. The testimonial segments I share with each Sanskrit mantra included in the book are gleaned from experiences of my clients after they've chanted specific mantras.

With a master's degree in psychology and a deep understanding of how the psyche operates, I've seen many clients become trapped in repetitive patterns, struggling to break through mental and emotional blocks. That's why I emphasize the psychological power of mantras – they offer a profound tool for calming the mind and clearing subconscious patterns that often cloud clarity and hinder the manifestation of goals.

Like Namadeva's work, this book is a practical application of Sanskrit mantras for seekers of spiritual solutions to everyday issues. Namadeva also taught mantras with an emphasis on practicality and efficiency as a tool in solving life problems. The aim of this book is to do the same. Namadeva would say that "the best mantra for you is the one you will actually do." He taught and explained mantras in a way that would be easy for Westerners to digest and practice. As it has been almost 20 years since Namadeva last published a book, I am hoping the continue in his tradition of making Sanskrit mantras easily accessible to those who want to enhance their self actualization process. This content can help to solve the problems that people contend with in current times in 21st century America, and the rest of the world. My background in psychology has helped me navigate the landscape of clients' subconscious and conscious issues while empowering them by providing a technique they can implement.

I am not writing this as a spiritual treatise, although I am versed in various Vedic scriptures as well as the importance and significance of the deities of the Hindu Pantheon, specifically as they relate to certain mantras. The profound spiritual wisdom of Sanskrit mantras – and the divine forms they embody – has been beautifully articulated in the extraordinary body of work by Sadguru Sant Keshavadas and his disciple, Namadeva Acharya.

I humbly bring my own experience of chanting in Sanskrit, teaching hundreds of workshops on Sanskrit mantras, and sharing them one-on-one with students and clients as remedies for their issues, as the qualifications for writing this book. I have gained wisdom on the application and efficacy of Sanskrit mantras through chanting them on a daily basis for 30+ years (and likely also in previous lifetimes). As a long-time professional consulting Western Astrologer, and more recently a Vedic Astrologer, I have seen the positive effects of recommending Sanskrit mantra remedies for difficult astrological aspects in one's natal chart or by transiting planets to the natal chart.

How Mantras Found Me

I wasn't seeking mantras – they found me. What unfolded was an unexpected and profound evolution, one that would eventually lead me to become a Certified Mantra Instructor many years after my first encounter with Sanskrit.

My introduction to Sanskrit mantras coincided with my first **Saturn Return** – that powerful astrological threshold when Saturn completes its orbit and returns to its natal position, between the ages of 28 to 30. At the time, I had already been working as a professional Western Astrologer for several years. So when both Yoga and Sanskrit mantras entered my life during this deeply karmic period, I understood the significance. It felt as though some past-life residue had risen to the surface, as if I were remembering ancient teachings embedded in the very fabric of my soul.

I had been regularly attending yoga classes several times a week at the Dhyanyoga Ashram in Connecticut, while I was working as a high school teacher. One day, the yoga instructor announced that the Guru of the lineage would be visiting the ashram – and that we had the rare opportunity to receive a spiritual initiation from her, known as *shaktipat*. The guru was Shri Anandi Ma, spiritual heir of the great Indian master Shri Dhyanyogi Madhusudandas. At the time, she was known as Asha Ma. Like Gurumayi Chidvilasananda, who succeeded Swami Muktananda, Asha Ma was one of the rare women appointed to carry a powerful spiritual lineage.

I was filled with anticipation as I prepared to receive *shaktipat* initiation from Shri Anandi Ma, the living representative of the unbroken Dhyanyoga lineage of Kundalini Maha Yoga. This lineage is distinct from **Kundalini Yoga** as taught by Yogi Bhajan.

I arrived at the ceremony with quiet reverence. As Asha Ma and her husband Dileepji chanted ancient Sanskrit mantras, something in me cracked open. I entered an altered state, and had a spontaneous past-life regression, slipping into a vivid vision of myself in a temple in India, chanting before flickering oil lamps. My spine felt like it was on fire, yet it was not painful – rather, it was alive with waves of energy, surging through my body in blissful currents.

When I returned to ordinary awareness, I couldn't remember a single mantra, yet I knew something in me had irrevocably shifted. Years later, I learned one of those mantras was the Bhuta Shuddhi Shringatat – a sacred key for awakening **kundalini** during *shaktipat.*

I was given a personal mantra: the Hanuman Chalisa – prescribed to help me navigate the karmic weight of Saturn during my Saturn Return. The instruction was clear: chant it 11 times a day for 40 days to clear **karma**.

The irony wasn't lost on me. At 28, just beginning my mantra path, I was handed a 40-verse hymn – complex, lengthy, and anything but beginner-friendly. Overwhelmed, I put it aside until I heard Krishna Das chant it in 2002. It wasn't until 2012 that I finally completed the full 40-day practice. In the meantime, my mystical mantra journey had already begun to unfold in its own mysterious rhythm.

Despite my hesitation with chanting the lengthy Hanuman Chalisa, I still was seeking to learn more about Sanskrit mantras. My path eventually led me to the short form of the Gayatri mantra, which I was introduced to through the Sai Baba lineage. A few friends and I began chanting it regularly together, and that's when my life began to shift – swiftly and profoundly.

As I committed to chanting the Gayatri mantra daily, subtle transformations began to unfold. Incredibly, within 18 months of starting my Gayatri practice, I had met my future husband, gotten married, and given birth to my son. This alone felt miraculous, especially because I had previously been told by doctors that I likely couldn't conceive due to a health condition that had manifested years earlier. By all medical accounts, my son's birth shouldn't have been possible – yet here he was. A true blessing, perhaps even a soul contracted to arrive through mantra and grace. The Gayatri mantra became the core of my spiritual practice, a sacred current I could ride each day.

In 1995 I received an in-person Vedic Astrology reading from the renowned Vedic Astrologer Chakrapani Ullal. He told me I had unlocked positive past-life karma through chanting Sanskrit mantras and urged me to reconnect more deeply with that sacred soul gift.

Fast forward to 2002: while browsing at Barnes & Noble, a book – *Healing Mantras* by Thomas Ashley-Farrand – quite literally flew off the shelf in front of me. I devoured it in just a few hours, completely captivated by the palpable energy and power radiating from its pages. Then, in a beautiful twist of synchronicity, a client gifted me the *Mantra: Sacred Words of Power* cassette series and study guide by the same author. She said she hadn't been able to connect with it and felt compelled to pass it on to me. I was floored. I listened to those tapes over and over, memorizing every mantra with devotion. I especially loved the longer "freight train mantras" like the Long Form Gayatri, the Apadamapa Mantra, and the Saraswati Maha Vidya Mantra. The experience completely blew my mind – and opened my heart.

After discovering *Healing Mantras*, I made a vow: I would meet Thomas Ashley-Farrand in person and become his mantra student.

There have been four key moments in my life when I felt so profoundly impacted by a spiritual teacher's work that I was determined to meet them and study under their guidance. These teachers were: visionary astrologer and author Barbara Hand Clow; psychic researcher and hypnosis pioneer Dick Sutphen; mantra master Thomas Ashley-Farrand; and my Vedic astrology guru Komilla Sutton.

Barbara Hand Clow was the first. Her early books – *Chiron* and *The Liquid Light of Sex* – sparked a deep awakening in me in the early 1990s. Her later works on galactic consciousness, including *The Pleiadian Agenda* and *Alchemy of Nine Dimensions*, expanded my awareness even further. I met Barbara and her husband, Gerry Clow, in the mid-1990s. When they came to Massachusetts, I attended all their workshops. They later invited me to serve as a healer in their *Alchemy of Nine Dimensions* activation workshops.

In 2002, I met Dick Sutphen and his wife Tara at the New Frontiers Café in Sedona. They invited me to Dick's past-life regression seminar that evening. The experience was powerful – an energetic transmission that catalyzed a profound mystical unfolding over the months that followed.

Years later, in 2018, I attended the Sedona Vedic Astrology Conference and took a workshop with Komilla Sutton. I instantly recognized her as my Vedic Astrology teacher. I went on to study with her for four years, completing her certification program. In 2023, I was honored to be invited as a presenter in her esteemed international seminar: Fresh Talents of Vedic Astrology.

In 2005, I discovered that Thomas Ashley-Farrand would be teaching a mantra workshop in Cambridge, Massachusetts. I attended without hesitation. The moment I heard his voice I was awestruck. The vibration of his chanting filled the room with palpable energy. After the workshop, one of the organizers asked if I'd like to receive Gayatri initiation from him. I responded with an enthusiastic yes.

Namadeva performed a sacred ceremony to initiate me into the long form of the Gayatri mantra. As he chanted, I felt my third eye burst open with light. He also gave me specific mantra prescriptions based on my spiritual questions and life concerns – personal guidance that struck me to the core.

I soon learned he returned annually to the Boston area and to Kripalu in western Massachusetts. I became a devoted student, attending every workshop I could – bringing along clients and students who were equally captivated by his teachings. The Kripalu retreats were especially powerful, held in the resonance-rich space of a former ashram – perfect for deep mantra immersion.

Namadeva's student community was full of kindred spirits. I met Raji Gretchen Carmel, who hosted him at The Yoga Space in Keene, New Hampshire – a place I often brought my own students. After Namadeva's passing, Raji has continued his legacy through a certified mantra teacher training program and we still collaborate together. Bill Barry and his wife Denise were avid devotees, who also continue Namadeva's tradition of teaching mantras.

Several others carried the torch as well: Ravi Hegarty and Lisa Derosiers of Solar Dynasty Kirtan, and Larisa Stow of Shakti Tribe *kirtan* band. I introduced my student Shivani Silvia Sune and her daughter Lalita Laura Antunes to Namadeva. Shivani went on to share Sanskrit mantra teachings on YouTube, while Lalita blossomed into a *kirtan* performer.

In the summer of 2007, I joined Namadeva's retreat in the Sierra Madre Mountains of California. It was life-changing. There, I experienced the blazing power of the solar mantras – my solar plexus ignited with light. I met his wife, Satyabhama, and many of his West Coast devotees. The retreat culminated in a five-hour Sudarshana Chakra ceremony, where we chanted continuously before a sacred fire. I felt myself lifted into higher dimensions, surrounded by seekers, and carried by the transmission of this extraordinary mantra master.

From 2006 to 2010, I followed Namadeva's teachings wherever I could – retreats in Keene, Kripalu, and his temple near Portland, Oregon. It was there I witnessed his **Guru Diksha** ceremony with Guru Rama Mata. Her blessing remains etched in my soul.

At Kripalu, I attended the legendary five-day workshop which we devotees dubbed fondly as the "**Puja** Palooza," an event so potent that, nearly two decades later, we still speak of the energy that surged through the gathering – mystical, alive, unforgettable.

I hosted Namadeva's workshops in my yogic community of Cohasset, Massachusetts, introducing his sacred sound teachings to my students and friends. His presence left a lasting imprint on our community. At the time, we didn't realize those years were soon drawing to a close.

In 2010, he asked me to organize a major event in Boston. I rallied my *shakti* and organized a three-day celebration at the Sri Radha Bhakti Mandir in Holbrook, Massachusetts, featuring Namadeva, Satyabhama, Guru Rama Mata, and Sri Muralidhar Pai. Devotees gathered from across New England to chant, sing, and receive *darshan*. It was a moment of divine orchestration – one I now see as the passing of the torch.

That same year, I traveled to Oregon for Namadeva's final event. In September, as his physical form declined, a few of us were called to his side. One by one, we received the Guru Jyoti (light of the Guru) – the final transmission of divine light from our Mantra Guru.

What I couldn't have known then was how deeply this would shape the years to come, as I continued his legacy by hosting events with Satyabhama, Guru Rama Mata, and Muraliji to teach in the Boston area, carrying forward the light he had kindled.

Namadeva was clear – both in life and in Spirit – that I was to carry forward the mantra tradition through this book. When 2025 arrived, his message became urgent: *Complete it by the 15th anniversary of my Mahasamadhi – October 1, 2025.* This book is not just a continuation of Namadeva's legacy, but a transmission of his work, echoing through sacred sound into the future.

Ancient Sound Formulas for the New Age of Frequency

This book sets itself apart from those of my predecessors by serving as a vehicle to transmit ancient sound frequencies that are meant to catalyze ascension on the planet at this pivotal time. Earth is not merely a physical world, but a sentient being, Gaia, who is undergoing a profound evolutionary transformation. Many spiritual traditions and mystics speak of this era as a dimensional shift, a movement from third-dimensional density into the higher vibrational states of fourth and fifth-dimensional consciousness. These realms are characterized by Unity consciousness, the choice of love over fear, and the power of resonance over control. Humanity is being called to align with universal frequencies of peace, compassion, authenticity, and integrity – anchoring a more awakened and harmonious state of being on Earth.

We are living in a time defined by frequency and vibration. Consciousness is no longer viewed as a mere byproduct of the brain, but as a vast, intelligent field that we can access and transmit. As more beings awaken, turning inward through meditation, healing ancestral wounds, and dissolving limiting beliefs, they elevate their personal vibration. This individual refinement contributes to what many call the collective ascension – the great awakening of humanity.

Practices like Sanskrit mantra, sound healing, and astrology are ancient vibrational technologies returning to prominence now because they help us attune to cosmic rhythms and the music of the spheres. As the sages have long taught: *The universe does not respond to what you want. It responds to who you are – your frequency.* In these times, aligning your vibration through devotion, creativity, healing, sound, silence, and selfless service becomes more than personal transformation. It becomes an offering – a sacred act of planetary stewardship.

As I bring Sanskrit mantras into the context of our modern world, I welcome the reader into a carefully cultivated field, one shaped over years of study, practice, and experience, and rooted in traditions that also align with emerging understandings of energy and the quantum field. This book is designed to demonstrate the vibrational power of mantra in a direct and experiential way, going beyond intellectual analysis. It offers practical tools for integrating sacred sound into daily life as a means of self-awareness, healing, and personal growth.

I carry deep respect for the lineage and teachings I've been fortunate to learn from, and I share them here with humility and care. The reader is invited to explore mantra as a pathway to connect with their own inner wisdom and clarity. Think of this book not just as text on a page, but as a dynamic and interactive resource – a living energy field of sound and intention that supports transformation from the inside out. It is a vibrational gateway, a field encoded with frequencies passed through sacred transmission. As you read, chant, or simply sit with these sound formulas, you are invited to enter a direct relationship with the soul, the Source, and the unseen lineage behind the mantras.

Mantras can be considered as soul medicine, spiritual light compressed into sound form. The syllables are seeds of divinity planted in consciousness. The mantras are not mine. They are echoes of a divine intelligence that has been lovingly passed from teacher to student across the centuries. I have received them in the sacred context of oral initiation, and I share them not as inventions, but as living inheritances.

If this book has found you, it may be because you have chanted these sounds before, in other lives, other forms. Trust what you feel. You are not just learning mantras, you are reclaiming your role as a vehicle of sacred sound.

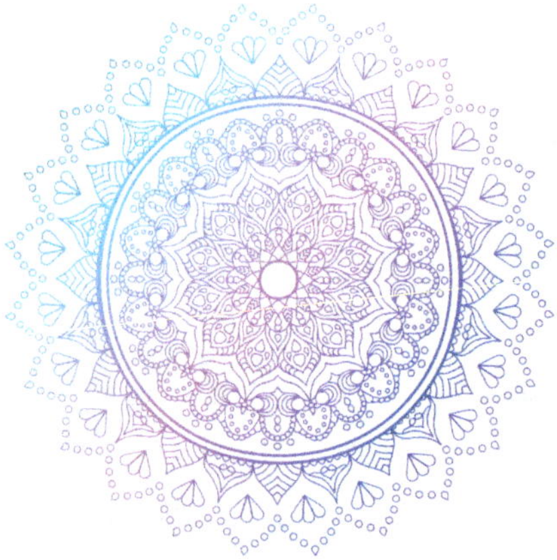

Psychological Blocks

We all tend to experience times in our life when we feel blocked or just can't seem to move forward. We may have the best intentions and work really hard toward our goals, but still feel like we aren't making headway.

There are seasons in life when progress feels blocked, and these periods can be frustrating, disheartening, even deeply discouraging. I've seen it often with clients – when nothing seems to move forward, it's tempting to slip into a victim mindset, convinced the world is against you and that luck has abandoned you. Be mindful – falling into victim mode only amplifies the sense that life is conspiring against you. Instead, choose to shift your perspective and consciously cultivate optimism. Hold the knowing that when the timing aligns, the path will open, the breakthrough will come, and you'll move forward with renewed momentum toward your success.

There are always reasons behind being blocked. Some may be obvious – such as health challenges, fatigue, or major life changes – while others dwell beneath the surface, hidden in the subconscious as an inner saboteur. At times, external influences – whether people or circumstances – may be slowing your growth. Other times, individuals, driven by envy, may quietly work to undermine your success – whether through negative speech, harmful intentions, or even use of darker energetic practices. Such actions disregard the immutable laws of karma, for any malice or ill will sent toward another inevitably returns to its source, magnified many times over.

Astrology & Right Timing

One of astrology's greatest gifts is teaching us how to align with the right timing. You may have the best intention to launch a new project or business, but the astrological alignments may not be working in your favor. This is especially true when someone tries to begin something during Mercury retrograde or an eclipse cycle, which tend to affect everyone and create obstacles in getting things off the ground.

We also experience times when our personal chart is under affliction from Saturn transiting our natal planets, creating blockages and challenges. Saturn, the taskmaster and lord of karma, arrives to help us pay karmic debts and sometimes learn tough lessons. Yet Saturn's ultimate purpose is to help us evolve by teaching mastery of ourselves and our karma. When Saturn hits, we must repeat the lesson until we understand what it's trying to teach.

Pluto is another archetype that pushes transformation, often taking us through death and birth initiations to reach the alchemical gold of healing. Pluto reveals hidden psychological wounds and the subconscious saboteur that blocks success.

Many people hold a deep fear of success, cycling through old patterns because they subconsciously resist change or fear what success or wealth might bring. I have guided many clients through this hidden fear, rooted in beliefs that success leads to loss, betrayal, or persecution.

These fears may stem from childhood experiences – seeing parents endure financial loss or reputational harm – or from soul memories carried across lifetimes, such as persecution for spiritual gifts or being on the "wrong" side of history after a power shift.

Others struggle with a fear of failure that keeps them from growth. Unlike fear of success, fear of failure arises from not meeting personal or external standards, often established in childhood when parents' expectations felt impossible to meet.

Whether obstacles stem from subconscious patterns, interference from others, or challenging astrological influences, these blockages can be cleared. With dedicated energy practices, it is possible to release these barriers and restore the flow toward your goals.

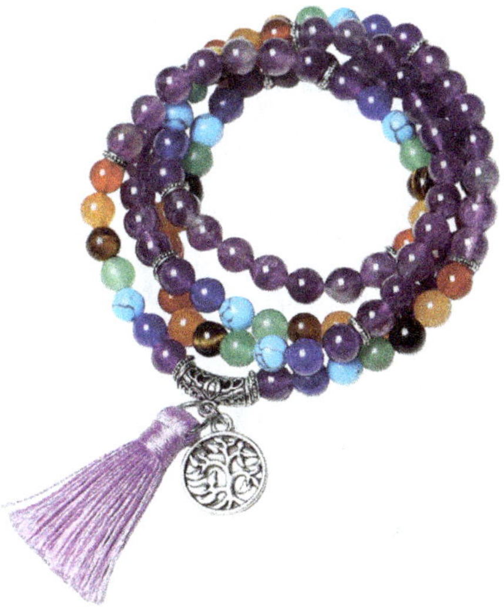

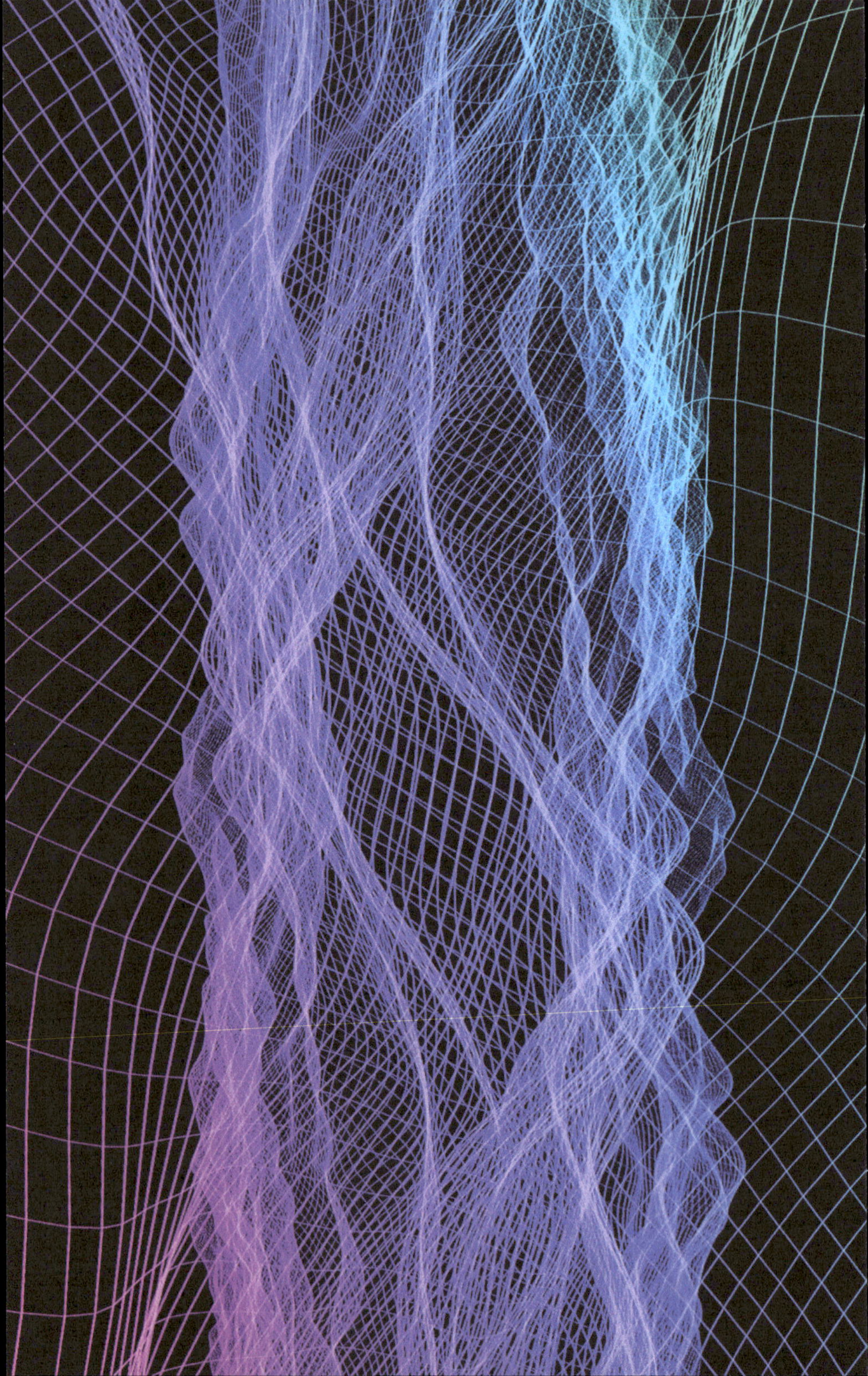

I

important concepts

Several key factors enhance the effectiveness of mantra chanting, helping it generate more positive results.

power of frequency

The famous quote by the inventor Nikola Tesla, "If you want to find the secrets of the universe, think in terms of energy, frequency, and vibration," is finally being understood by those bringing in the new paradigm of healing, which includes using light technology and vibrational medicine. Sanskrit Mantra Chanting is an ancient sound technology that works through energy, vibration, and frequency. As a vibrational language, its power arises from the energetic impact of the sounds released when chanted. Pronouncing a mantra creates a particular physical vibration in the form of sound. The sound vibration generates distinct effects in both the physical body and **subtle body**. These specific energetic impacts are understood as the very meaning of the mantra that produces them. In essence, the true power of a mantra lies not in its literal Sanskrit translation, but in the transformative effect its repeated sound vibrations have on the person chanting it. Sanskrit is a vibrational language which resonates at a frequency that is higher than other spoken words or sounds.

Our energetic vibration creates our reality. As the **Buddha** said, "We do not see the world as it is. *Rather, we see the world as we are.*" The habitual ego thoughtforms that typically make up most of our conscious mental experience frame our world and direct our attention. Accordingly, we then either successfully or unsuccessfully recognize opportunities and threats in our surroundings. Unrecognized opportunities cannot help us and imagined threats can torment us, so it is imperative that we are able to align more effectively with reality as it is, without the cloud of illusion that our mind habitually traffics in (called **maya** in Sanskrit).

Our mental patterns can be thought of as vibrational frequencies. Lower vibrations bind us to illusion and suffering; higher vibrations free us, aligning us with the higher dimensional reality always available but seldom recognized. Sanskrit mantras call upon the highest frequencies of the universe and connect us with the life current of divinity. The Book of John opens, "In the beginning was the Word, and the Word was with God, and the Word was God." The Vedic tradition of ancient India agrees – the Word is **Om**.

Sound healing has become popular in yoga and holistic spaces, using crystal bowls, Tibetan bowls, drums, and gongs. I was trained as a gong healer and use it to clear and raise vibration at the end of classes or workshops. When sound healing is applied, it offers many benefits to students. Chanting Sanskrit mantras produces the same effects – except the only instrument needed is one's own voice. You become the instrument and feel the vibration move through the body.

The gong and Sanskrit chanting enhance healing by creating space for the mind to release and the subconscious to clear. Both work through the body's subtle energy pathways – the **nadis** in Sanskrit and meridians in Chinese medicine – softening blocks, improving circulation, and reducing tension. Emotional transformation follows as sound reorganizes energy within the body and calms the nervous system. Our **chakras** – energetic gateways linked to the glands – align and activate, supporting greater awareness and expanded consciousness.

When the gong is played with proper technique and mantras are articulated with precise pronunciation, they generate coherent vibrational patterns that facilitate the synchronization of neural pathways, thereby promoting optimal physiological function. Conversely, practitioners lacking adequate training or expertise in sound healing may inadvertently produce dissonant or incoherent frequencies, which can lead to adverse effects such as headaches and other symptoms. As sound healing has entered the mainstream, many individuals claim expertise in playing the gong or other sound instruments without proper training, which can sometimes result in causing more harm than healing. The transmission of mantras through an experienced teacher ensures the preservation of their authentic vibrational integrity, safeguarding against incoherence and maintaining their therapeutic efficacy as established within traditional lineages.

Part of what makes mantra chanting so effective is its tangible energetic impact on the body. My teacher, Namadeva, explained, "This is because mantras are composed of chakra-based sounds. Each of the fifty letters in the Sanskrit alphabet corresponds to one of the fifty petals found across the first six chakras, from the base of the spine up to the brow center. The sacred Vedic texts known as the **Upanishads** describe how advanced spiritual **adepts** possess the ability to actually see the Sanskrit letters inscribed on the petals of the chakras."*

Namadeva explained further, "When a Sanskrit mantra is spoken, the corresponding petals on the chakras vibrate in spiritual resonance. This activates and energizes each petal, tuning it to a higher frequency. As a result, ambient spiritual energy in the surrounding space is drawn toward the individual chanting the mantra."**

In this way, mantras influence both the physical body and the spiritual consciousness – we grow not only in spirit, but also in form. In addition to our minds, our physical bodies also benefit from the positive vibrational impact of Sanskrit

* Thomas-Ashley Farrand, *Teacher of Mantra Instruction Manual* (Saraswati Publications, 2008), 80.
** Ibid., 81.

mantras. By chanting mantras, we can help manifest our desired outcomes by drawing them into tangible form.

Mantras have only approximate translations in spoken language; their true meaning lies in the experience they evoke within the individual who chants them. From the original **seer** or creator to the many who have chanted it since, each mantra gains an "experiential definition" – it is known by the specific energetic effect it produces. For example, the **Lakshmi** mantra "Om Shrim Maha Lakshmiyei Namaha" calls upon Lakshmi, the Goddess of Prosperity. It is chanted to attract abundance or to cultivate a felt sense of trust that one's needs are being fulfilled. This was the original energetic impression received by the seer, and it has continued to resonate with practitioners throughout the ages.

Chanting Sanskrit mantras activates and amplifies **prana**, the vital life force that underlies all functions of the body and mind – breathing, circulation, digestion, movement, and thought. While *prana* flows through the physical body, it is not physical itself; it belongs to the subtle body. Remarkably, *prana* can be consciously transferred between individuals – some healers work through the intentional transmission of this energy. Self-healing is also possible by directing *prana* to a specific organ. When a mantra is chanted while visualizing an internal organ bathed in light, the vibrational power of the mantra can become focused in that area, bringing profound and beneficial effects.

power of intention

The power of intention is frequently mentioned in discussions about manifestation philosophies, spiritual practices, and New Age thought. In this context, intention refers to the ability of a focused and purposeful thought to influence energy, behavior, and outcomes – both within ourselves and in the external world. In spiritual and energetic traditions, intention is considered the guiding force behind action, manifestation, and transformation. Some of the aspects of conscious intention is the way it can channel energy focusing the mind and *prana* toward a specific goal, whether for healing, clarity, or manifestation.

Intention is a bridge between thought and reality and therefore the seed of creation. As the adage goes: "energy flows where attention goes." Whatever we hold our awareness on with mental clarity begins to shape our inner experience, and over time our external world.

When chanting a mantra, meditating, visualizing, or engaging in any spiritual discipline, intention magnifies the result. A mantra chanted mindlessly is different from one infused with heartfelt purpose. Intention gives spiritual practices depth, direction, and potency. Pure intention – rooted not in ego or desire, but in alignment with truth or higher purpose – carries transformative power. In many traditions it is believed that when intention aligns with the divine, the universe cooperates in unseen ways.

When chanting Sanskrit, it is advised to set an intention, or **sankalpa**. *Sankalpa* is seen as the invisible current that directs the sound vibration. The mantra is the vehicle; intention is the driver. The clearer and more sincere the intent, the more precise and powerful the energetic effect.

When the physical sound vibration of a mantra is combined with the mental force of intention, the energetic impact of the mantra is greatly amplified. Intention – the purpose behind the chanting – rides on the vibration of the sound, directing its power toward a specific effect. This union of sound and intent is the very essence of Sanskrit.

Ultimately, chanting Sanskrit mantras calms the mind. The word mantra derives from Sanskrit words *manas*, which means mind, and *trai*, which means to protect or set free from. Etymologically, the word mantra means "to free from the mind." A mantra is a mental tool, capable of liberating us from conditioned psychological patterns and the limitations of preordained circumstances. Everyone engages in a continuous stream of inner dialogue, composed of automatic thoughts that may arise consciously or operate at a subconscious level. This mental chatter often persists whether we are fully aware of it or not. Most individuals exert little control over the ruminative patterns of their mind, which can subtly yet powerfully shape the course of their lives. For example, a woman who steps on the scale each morning and thinks, "I'm too fat; I need to lose weight," is feeding her mind a recurring thought that begins to dominate her inner narrative. This internalized belief may resurface throughout the day – guiding her eating choices, compelling her to exercise, or reinforcing self-critical behaviors. Over time, the thoughtform of being overweight becomes a defining lens through which she experiences reality. Unless consciously addressed – through practices such as affirmations or mantra – this pattern can continue to govern her perception and behavior.

Affirmations are often compared to mantras as tools for reshaping subconscious patterns. I said affirmations for many years before discovering Sanskrit mantras. However, affirmations spoken in the speaker's native language may lack the intrinsic vibrational qualities of traditional mantras.

From a psychological and neuroscientific perspective, this can lead to cognitive dissonance – where the subconscious mind resists or contradicts affirmations that conflict with deeply held beliefs. For example, a person striving to cultivate prosperity consciousness might repeat affirmations such as, "I am wealthy, I am prosperous, I have plenty of money." Yet, if their subconscious remains influenced by early experiences of scarcity and poverty, neural pathways associated with these limiting beliefs can trigger resistance, blocking the affirmation from being fully integrated. This reflects how established neural circuits and implicit memory can undermine conscious intentions, highlighting the importance of approaches that engage the brain's plasticity to effectively rewire these patterns.

Research indicates that chanting mantra generates specific vibrational frequencies that can modulate brainwave activity and influence subconscious neural pathways. This process promotes neuroplasticity, enabling the brain to rewire entrenched thought patterns and reduce habitual mental rumination, ultimately facilitating cognitive and emotional transformation.*

The proverb "As a man thinketh, so is he" (Proverbs 23:7) means that a person's inner thoughts and attitudes shape their outward actions and overall character. The phrase reflects a core psychological truth. Our internal thought patterns significantly shape our perception, behavior, and life outcomes. By fostering constructive and affirmative thinking, we can positively influence our emotional well-being, relationships, and overall life trajectory. The good news is that chanting mantras can shift the subconscious patterns of thought and mind ramblings by vibrations which literally override these old patterns.

When practiced consistently over an extended period, mantra possesses the capacity to subdue the fragmented and incoherent patterns of the subconscious mind. Much like a dominant waveform subsumes a lesser one, the rhythmic

* Aviva Berkovich-Ohana, et al, "Repetitive Speech Elicits Widespread Deactivation in the Human Cortex: The 'Mantra' Effect?" *Brain and Behavior* 5, no. 7 (2015): e00346. https://doi.org/10.1002/brb3.346

repetition of mantra overrides the fluctuations of random thoughtforms. With disciplined practice, mantra can penetrate deeply embedded cognitive imprints – often held somatically in the organs and glands – transmuting these physiological centers into vessels of tranquility. Repetitive ruminations can be ceased and the mind becomes calm. The subconscious no longer holds the dominant control of one's life. It is commonly said that the subconscious mind governs 90-95% of our mental activity, while the conscious mind makes up only 5-10%. This estimate is widely cited in psychology and neuroscience to illustrate how much of our behavior, habits, decisions, and perceptions are driven by unconscious processes.*

After chanting enough mantras, the subconscious becomes integrated with the conscious mind, thus giving us conscious direction over our mind and essentially enhancing our free will. It can then become a supportive channel – offering insight through dreams and psychic impressions that are free from ego distortion. Initially, this shift may create a sense of mental emptiness or disorientation, as familiar thought patterns quiet down. However, this space allows the higher mind – rooted in intellect and intuition – to take the lead, guiding the individual toward a more balanced and conscious way of living.

* Robert Williams, "Processing Information with the Nonconscious Mind," *Journal Psyche*, https://journalpsyche.org/processing-information-with-nonconscious-mind

about ancient vedic teachings

The **Vedas**, the world's oldest scriptures and the sacred texts of Hinduism, are the first known source of Sanskrit mantras. The Vedas include the *Rig Veda*, *Sama Veda*, *Yajur Veda*, and *Atharva Veda*. The Vedas teach that every being is composed of the five elements – earth, water, fire, air, and ether. In deep meditation, the ancient sages (*rishis*) perceived the subtle interplay of sound vibrations underlying these elemental forces. From these insights, they discerned and recorded the 50-letter Sanskrit alphabet as a reflection of these cosmic patterns. Through careful observation and inner vision, they came to understand how specific sound combinations – mantras – resonate with and influence the fabric of the universe. Because of their profound perception and the practical application of these sound formulas, they became known as the *seers of mantras*.

Vedic mantras were primarily used in rituals such as **yagnas** (fire ceremonies) and offerings to invoke gods, natural forces, and universal principles. They were considered sound embodiments of divine energy.

Following the Vedas, additional scriptures emerged: the **Brahmanas**, the Aranyakas, and the **Upanishads**. The Brahmanas delve into the details of ritual practice but focus primarily on the deeper meaning and significance behind those rituals. The Aranyakas, often called the "forest treatises," were intended for sages and practitioners living in seclusion, offering rituals and meditative reflections suited to solitary life. These texts also include teachings on the term Brahmana, referring not only to the ritual specialist but also to the creative power inherent in ritual – a power believed to sustain and align with the cosmic order.

The Upanishads revolve around the intimate act of gathering around a teacher for spiritual instruction and inner inquiry. These texts gave rise to a body of profound philosophical literature that explores themes such as self-realization, yoga, meditation, karma, and reincarnation. At their core, the Upanishads were composed to sustain and deepen reflection on life beyond death, while preserving the relevance of spiritual merit and the soul's journey. They serve as a bridge between ritual practice and inner wisdom, keeping alive essential questions about the nature of existence and the path to liberation.

The **Tantras** appeared later in Hindu scriptures and focused on practical methods for spiritual awakening. Unlike the Vedas, which emphasize ritual and sacrifice, the Tantras prioritize personal experience, inner transformation, and direct access to the divine through specific techniques. The Tantras emphasized mantra, *yantra*, and ritual, or using sacred sound, visual symbols, and ceremonies to awaken spiritual energy. It is from the Tantras that the idea of kundalini and chakras as detailed maps of the subtle body and energy centers emerged. The Tantras also emphasized deity worship especially focused on **Shiva**, **Shakti**, and other divine forms. The Tantras are considered esoteric and were traditionally taught in secrecy, often requiring initiation (*diksha*). They have significantly influenced Yoga, **Ayurveda**, mantra practice, and meditation traditions in both Hinduism and Buddhism.

In Tantra, mantras are not merely tools for attraction, but sacred vibrational codes that awaken the latent energies within. As you chant with focused intention and devotion, your inner *shakti* – the creative life force – is activated and begins to resonate with the cosmic patterns of existence. This heightened vibration aligns you with the subtle forces of the universe, drawing toward you what is in harmony with your evolving energetic state – whether that be a soul-aligned partner, purposeful work, or any experience that supports your spiritual unfolding. In this way, attraction is not manipulation, but the natural consequence of inner alignment with divine energy.

Mantras derive from other sources of Hindu scripture such as the **Puranas**, **Devi Bhagavatam**, and great Sutras including the **Yoga Sutras of Patanjali**.

In Vedic Astrology, one can chant the Vedic, Tantric, or Puranic mantra to help mitigate planetary karma. The Vedic planetary mantra is short and simple while the Tantric mantra includes seed sounds, making it more powerful. Puranic mantras are used to honor and appease the **Navagrahas**, or nine planetary deities in Vedic astrology.

These mantras are devotional in nature and typically invoke the grace, protection, and favorable influence of a specific planet.

Namadeva spoke to this connection of Sanskrit mantras and the transits of planets: "The movement of the planets through spheres of force and influence represented by the various signs and houses in one's astrological chart affect our lives in profound ways on a daily basis. Sanskrit mantras can change the way we receive those powerful vibrations. Secrets pertaining to the use of mantra in application to the natal astrological chart were kept hidden by the Brahmin priesthood for centuries."*

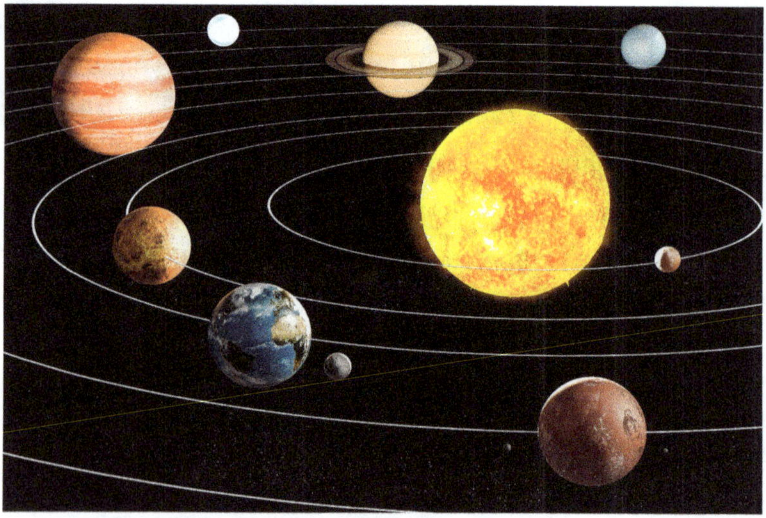

* Thomas Ashley-Farrand, *The Ancient Power of Sanskrit Mantra and Ceremony*, vol. 2 (Saraswati Publications, 2013), 122.

astrology and mantras

Skilled modern day Vedic Astrologers integrate Sanskrit mantras into their astrological practice by prescribing mantras as remedies for issues in a client's chart. An adept astrologer (from either the Vedic or Western astrological tradition) can quickly identify challenges and opportunities inherent in a client's chart by examining the client's natal chart and current transits or planetary phases that are currently impacting the client. Typically, favorably placed planets in a person's birth chart manifest as personal strengths and skills while unfavorably placed planets manifest as personal weaknesses or blind spots. Positive transits or planetary phases (called **dashas** in the Vedic system) tend to manifest as time periods of opportunity or good luck, while challenging transits or phases manifest as times rife with obstacles and challenges.

However, the unique advantage a competent Vedic Astrologer familiar with Sanskrit mantras has is that they are able to offer more than just guidance to their clients; *they are able to offer powerful energetic solutions through recommending mantra remedies.* For example, an astrologer might warn a client going through a challenging Mars cycle to be extra cautious, avoid risky situations and people, minimize conflicts and arguments, and be mindful of anger both within them and in their environment. Although such advice might be very valuable to help navigate the Mars cycle, the client's experience would be greatly enhanced if the astrologer also prescribed an appropriate mantra, perhaps one for the planet Mars itself or maybe a mantra invoking the energy of the spiritual warrior represented as **Hanuman**. Having the right mantra as a tool in one's spiritual toolbox could make the difference between a tough period of time filled with suffering, or an uplifting period filled with growth and opportunity.

Through mantra practice, a person can amplify the positive in their astrological chart, mitigate the negative, or both. Ultimately a person's astrological chart is a map of their personal karma and as mantras work directly with karma, they are an ideal remedy for astrological issues. It's a common belief among Vedic practitioners that "everything is karma," therefore mantras can help with everything. It is considered a great blessing to discover and be interested in the practice of Sanskrit mantras in one's life. It points to excellent karma from positive past action, in this life or a previous one. You, dear reader, can appreciate that by being someone reading this book you have such a blessing from your positive past actions. It is a further blessing to have the desire to pursue the mantra practice and also the discipline to follow through with it. Knowing which specific mantra to say to directly target your personal karma indicated in your astrological chart is an even greater blessing.

If you are deeply familiar with your own astrological chart then you might already know which planets would benefit from mantras. However, if you are not already an expert on your own astrological chart then it would be wise to seek the counsel of an experienced astrologer, including the authors of this book, who are both astrologers that implement Sanskrit mantras in their readings. They can help you navigate your planetary karmas by recommending an appropriate mantra for you.

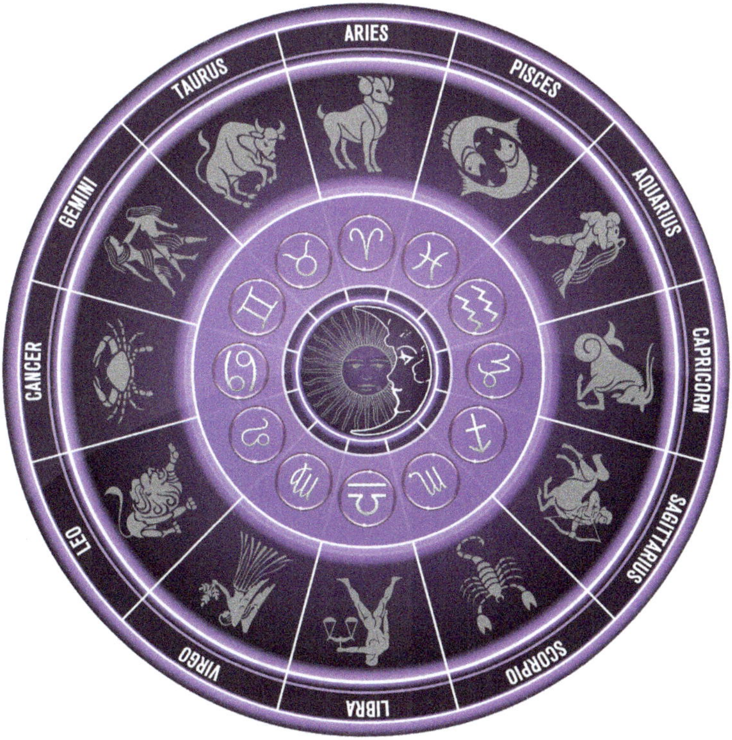

additional benefits of chanting mantras

When we chant Sanskrit mantras magical things can happen. We may feel warmth and healing moving through our bodies, illumination of consciousness, and/or other sensations. Chanting mantras offers countless benefits, many which activate unique responses within the individual. As the sacred sounds are repeated, the *nadis* begin to clear, often producing noticeable sensations. These can include tingling, the feeling of coolness or heat, a trickling or dripping sensation, waves of "spiritual goosebumps" or kundalini chills, or even the subtle impression of a light touch, like a spider or insect moving gently along the arm or leg.

Pay close attention to the sensations or subtle vibrations that arise during or after chanting, as they often reveal areas of the body or layers of emotion that are being cleared and realigned. It is common to experience vibrations or waves of heat, especially along the spine, in the heart center, or at the crown of the head. Other sensations may include tingling or a feeling of lightness or heaviness. *Kriyas*, or spontaneous movements, may emerge, such as gentle swaying or rocking, or even naturally moving into yogic postures, as the body releases and integrates the mantra's power.

During mantra chanting, one may notice shifts in the natural rhythm of the breath, sometimes slowing into deep stillness, at other times quickening with the flow of energy.

These altered breathing patterns are a natural response, as chanting helps to regulate the nervous system, quiet the mind, and awaken the movement of *prana*, the vital life force carried on the breath. Rhythmic chanting and breath regulation can lower heart rate, reduce blood pressure, and synchronize brainwave activity, all of which support mental clarity and emotional stability. Over time, chanting strengthens respiratory function, improves oxygenation in the body, and enhances overall vitality.

Chanting mantras can bring about profound mental and emotional shifts, often guiding the practitioner into a state of deep inner peace or heightened mental clarity. At times, the practice opens the heart to emotional release, which may arise as unexpected tears, waves of joy, or even moments of blissful ecstasy. Old patterns of anger, fear, or anxiety may also surface and dissolve, allowing the individual to experience a greater sense of freedom, balance, and emotional resilience.

Chanting mantras can also open the door to subtle sensory phenomena. Auditory experiences may arise, such as hearing tones, or inner sounds, or even a mantra repeating itself as though whispered into the ear. I have often heard the sounds of the *Gandarvas,* or celestial musicians, echoing the chant back from the unseen corners of the room. Visual impressions can occur, ranging from flashes of lights to **mandalas** or symbolic imagery that emerge with the inner vision. As the practice deepens, one may even experience distortions of time and space, slipping beyond the bounds of linear reality into a more expansive state of consciousness.

Many practitioners describe profound spiritual experiences arising from mantra chanting such as moments of deep unity with all that exists, and visions of spiritual beings, guides, or archetypal presences. At times sudden revelations or insights into the nature of self, reality, or divine truth may unfold. Such experiences often awaken greater compassion, patience, and inner strength, while forging a deeper spiritual connection and fostering a natural detachment from worldly concerns.

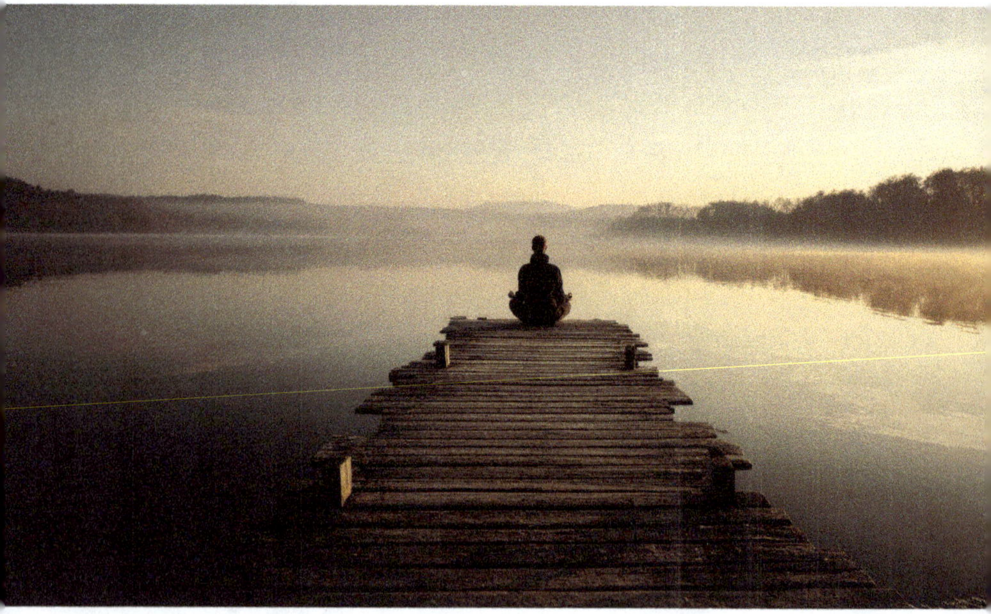

chakras, kundalini, and shakti

In order to understand how mantras work, it is essential to understand the Yogic Spiritual physiology that includes the concepts of chakras, **kundalini**, and **shakti**.

The actual translation of the Sanskrit word chakra is "wheel of light." The common use of the word chakra in modern day refers to energetic wheels within our subtle bodies. The spiritual chakras are spinning energy centers, or vortexes, of our subtle body that align with the major nerve ganglia along the spine of the physical body. Chakras are often described as flower-like in nature. When activated, some spiritual teachers liken them to radiant wildflowers, vibrant and full of life. Just as the nerve plexuses regulate our various bodily systems, the chakras continuously receive and distribute *prana* throughout both the physical and subtle bodies. According to Vedic physiology, there are seven major chakras in the body.

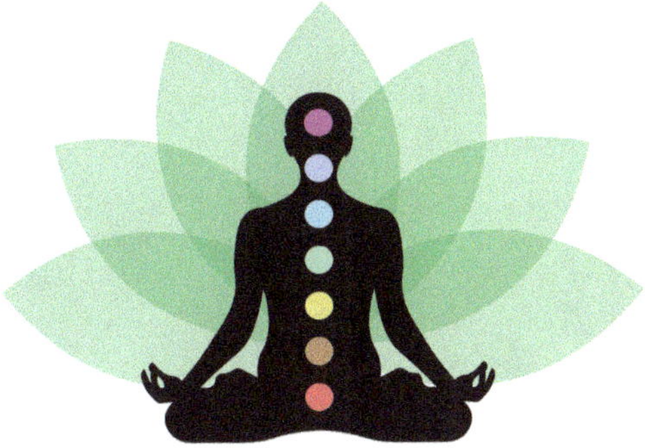

seed sounds
chakra bija mantras

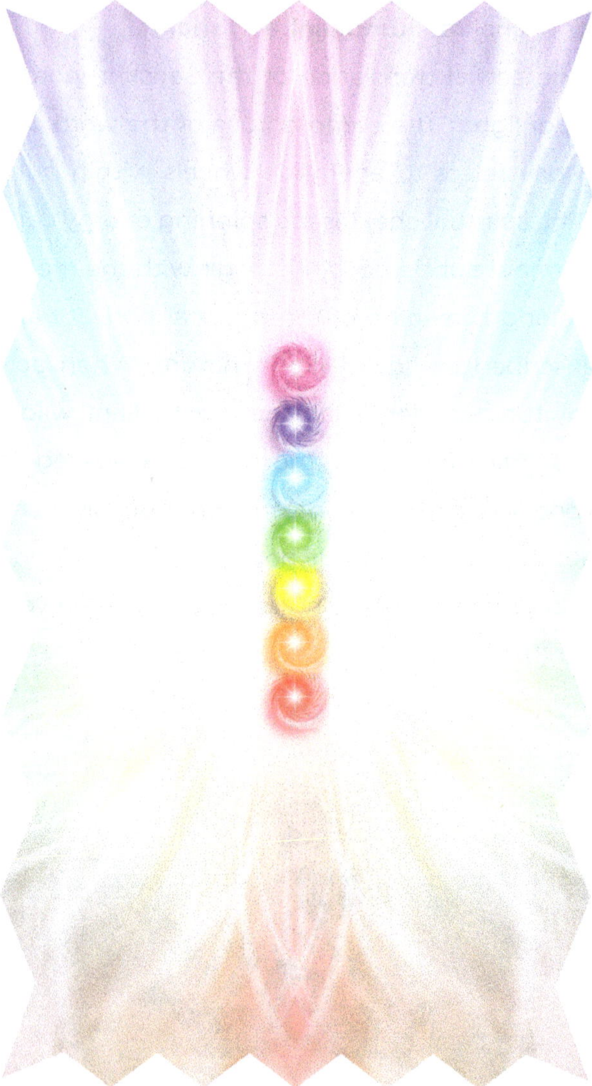

Each of the seven main chakras has a **bija mantra**, or seed mantra, that activates energy in that center. Chanting these chakra *bijas* prepares the chakras to move and process energy. The seed sound Ram stimulates the solar plexus, or third chakra – known as the body's healing or sun center – creating *tapas* (spiritual heat) that supports digestion and overall vitality. When the third chakra is activated, one may sense warmth or hear gurgling sounds as energy moves through the body. Here are the chakra *bijas*, beginning with the first chakra:

muladhara

Red | Root chakra | Earth
Base of spine
Stability, safety, survival and security, grounding, survival, safety

Lam (Lahm): This seed mantra activates the **Muladhara Chakra**, or first energy center located at the base of the spine. Lam brings attunement with the Earth principle. Lam adds the quality of spiritual scent or smell. Sometimes when one chants "Lam" they smell sandalwood or roses, symbolic of the presence of Divine Mother, in whatever form one relates to her. It could be signifying the presence of Mother Mary from the Christian tradition or Lakshmi or Durga in the Vedic pantheon.

svadhistana swadistha

Orange | Sacral chakra | Water
Lower abdomen (just below the navel)
Emotions, pleasure, rules digestion and assimilation, creativity, sexuality

Vam (Vahm): This seed mantra is for the **Swadisthana** chakra. Vam activates the watery principle and the attunement to spiritual taste. Often, when one chants "Vam," they may get a sweet taste in their mouth, which is nectar-like. This is actually a spiritual phenomenon of creating *amrita* (spiritual nectar) in the body. Chanting "Vam" can cause one to feel ravenous or hungry; it can tame too strong appetites and/or bring a greater sense of control for food, sex, and other sensual desires.

manipura

Yellow | Solar Plexus chakra | Fire
Upper abdomen (stomach area)
Power, confidence, body's healing center, personal power, willpower

Ram (Rahm): This *bija* sound is for the **Manipura** chakra, the third energy center, located in the solar plexus region. Ram brings attunement to the principle of fire, and creates *tapas* or spiritual heat in the body which can aid with digestion or burn through karma. Chanting "Ram" can help with digestion issues, or when one can't stomach something physically, emotionally, or energetically. It ignites the inner fire (digestive and spiritual), supports transformation and purification, and enhances willpower, confidence, and self-mastery.

anahata

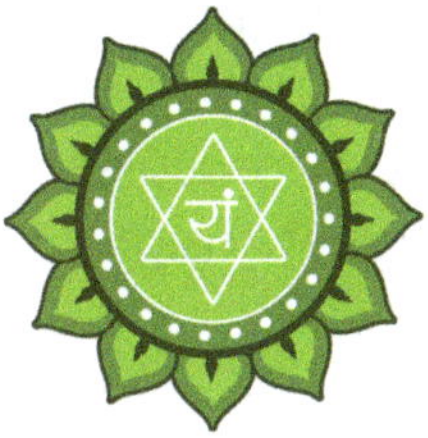

Green | Heart chakra | Air
Center of the chest
Love, compassion, quality of touch, forgiveness

Yam (Yahm): This *bija* mantra activates the **Anahata** chakra, or energy center located at the heart center. Yahm brings attunement with the principle of air, and rules the quality of touch. One may feel the touch of angels or divine beings when chanting "Yam." Chanting this mantra can help one hear the voices of divine beings, or celestial musicians called the *Gandarvas*. Chanting Yam can open the heart center, bringing more self-love and compassion. This simple seed mantra can help heal a broken heart.

vishuddha

Blue | Throat chakra | Akasha (Ether)
Neck and throat at the laryngeal and pharyngeal nerve plexus
Communication, truth, expression

Hum (Hum, like to "hum" a song): This seed sound is for the **Vishuddha** chakra located in the neck and throat. Hum brings attunement with the principle of *akasha*. Hum rules the quality of sound, and can help with hearing subtle sounds and frequencies. Chanting "Hum" can help one learn and understand Sanskrit mantras better, as well as learning other languages. Chanting "Hum" can assist in healing afflictions of the throat area, including thyroid and parathyroid issues.

ajna

Indigo | Third eye chakra | Light
Between the eyebrows
Intuition, vision, where the masculine and feminine currents meet, insight, imagination

Om (Ohm): Om is the seed sound for the **Ajna** chakra located in the third eye center. Om rules the cosmic mind, and connects to universal consciousness. Om brings attunement to the principle of Unity, and transcends polarity by bringing unity of integration of the pairs of opposites, such as male and female, or hot and cold, etc. Chanting "Om" can still the mind, and release worries and anxieties.

sahasrara

Violet | Crown chakra | Cosmic energy or Consciousness
Top of the head
Spiritual connection, enlightenment, connects to the subtle body and the soul

Silent Om: The silence after chanting "Om" activates the Sahasrara chakra, located at the crown of the head. The silence transcends sound and activates our personal **cosmic consciousness**, merging with the *purusha* (Universal Oversoul).

Some traditions associate the third eye chakra with violet and the crown chakra color as luminous white.

additional information on chakras

There are also chakras in the hands and feet. Many healers possess strongly activated hand chakras, and some people are born with them wide open. By engaging consistently in hands-on healing, chi practices such as qigong, tai chi, or hand yoga, one can open their hand chakras and increase the potency of energies flowing through them.

Some of the largest chakras in the body are located in the feet. These energy centers play a vital role in drawing in health-giving earth energy. They are naturally activated when we walk barefoot, establishing a direct connection with the earth. It is important to be grounded by walking in nature, or other earthing methods, to better embody the healing vibrations emitting from planet Earth. The Earth has its own pulsation described as "the heartbeat of Mother Earth," by indigenous peoples. This frequency is referred to as the "Schumann Resonance" by the scientific community. The Schumann Resonance refers to a set of low-frequency electromagnetic resonances that occur in the space between the Earth's surface and the ionosphere. These resonances are essentially like the Earth's "natural heartbeat" and are caused by lightning strikes that create electromagnetic waves which bounce around the Earth's atmosphere. The Schumann frequency is approximately 7.83 Hz, with additional resonances at 14.3, 20.8, 27.3 and 33.8 Hz. Those electromagnetic waves get trapped in the cavity between the Earth and the ionosphere and reverberate. These resonances provide a global "background" frequency for the Earth. They are used in research related to weather, climate, and even geophysical events like earthquakes.

On an energetic level, the Schumann frequency 7.83 Hz aligns closely with the alpha and beta brainwave states that are associated with relaxation, meditation, creativity, and dreaming. The Schumann Resonance upliftments provide a fascinating correlation to the results achieved by chanting Sanskrit mantras in attaining those brainwaves.

Earth changes and consciousness shifts over the past years have contributed to this increase in planetary pulsation. Some think that this spiking of the Schumann Resonance is accelerating an ascension process or vibrational shift in all species on Planet Earth including humans. This is experienced as time speeding up as well as humanity waking up to multi-dimensionality, or higher states of awareness, where emotional, physical, and spiritual awakenings occur more rapidly and frequently. The enhanced Schumann Resonance can also support kundalini awakening, energy healing, detoxification, cellular regeneration, and chakra activation, which are also the benefits of chanting Sanskrit mantras.

Once awakened and empowered by **kundalini shakti**, the foot chakras can also become channels for emitting energy. This energy may take the form of spiritual light, which can be directed in a narrow beam or dispersed more widely – guided by the conscious intention of one who is skilled in spiritual practice.

A spiritually potent current, alive, electric, and tangible, can be transmitted through touch. When a realized being permits another to touch their feet, they may become a living conduit, transmitting the radiant force of *shakti* with intention and grace.

Namadeva gave a profound example of this transmission in the story of Jesus washing the feet of his disciples – an act that can be seen as preparing their foot chakras to receive higher frequencies of divine energy or enhanced kundalini energies.

As it was described in the Upanishads, there flows a subtle fire, unseen yet all-pervading, that moves through the knower of the Divine. When the awakened one permits the touch of their feet, the sacred energy of *shakti* is not merely given – it arises, as dawn from night, as breath from stillness, and is imparted in silence more powerful than words.

Chanting sacred Sanskrit sound formulas activates *shakti*, which also represents the Divine Feminine life force. *Shakti* can be transmitted from gurus or teachers to students, from healers to receivers. These mantras can also mitigate negative planetary influences and enhance positive planetary aspects. Chanting helps to optimize health and well-being, calm the mind, and make one focused and relaxed. On esoteric levels, chanting in Sanskrit clears karma and removes *samskaras*. Chanting in Sanskrit activates kundalini *shakti*. Chanting also energizes the spiritual physiology of the chakras and subtle pathways of the *nadis*. Through chanting, one can attain **siddhi** (spiritual power) and **buddhi** (wisdom). Chanting in Sanskrit can clear the space internally or outside of you, such as in a room or home, and as a by-product uplift the physical environment.

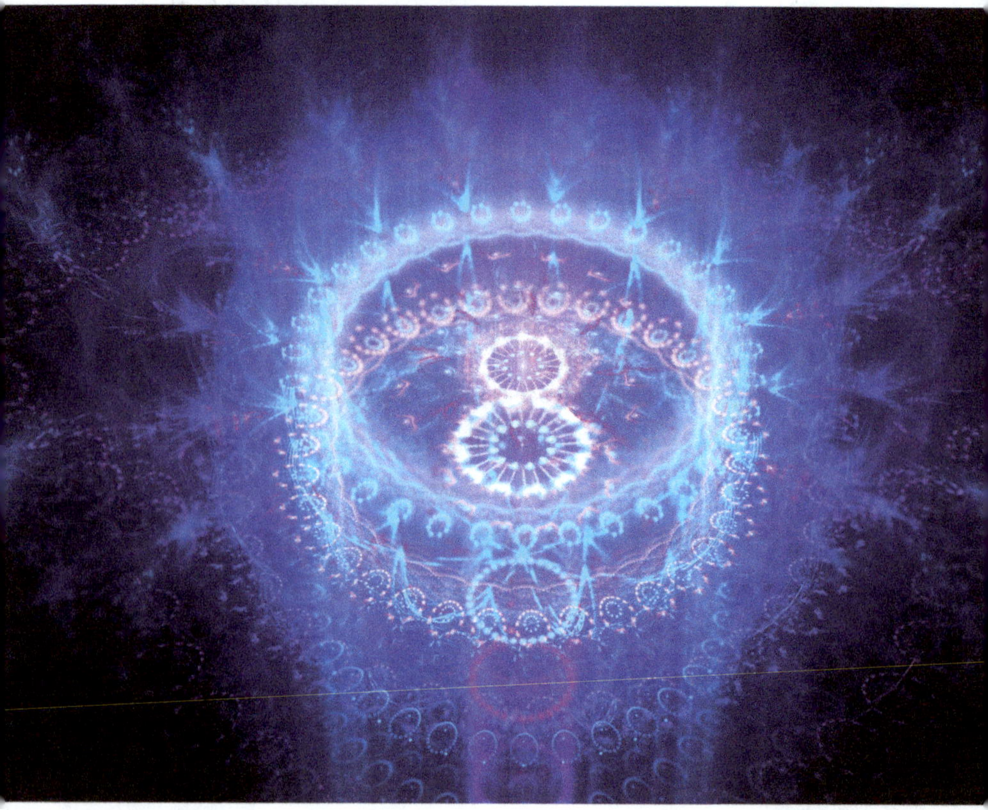

kundalini and shakti

The terms kundalini, Kundalini Shakti, and shakti are used interchangeably to describe the powerful life force that lies dormant at the base of the spine. This energy awakens as the individual becomes attuned to the power of their soul and the divine life force. Usually, it takes yogic, energetic, or spiritual interventions to spark kundalini. Kundalini is a powerful energy cell and transformative force located at the base of the spine. It is feminine in nature, and is inherently more active in women than in men. The energy of kundalini follows the path of our spiritual journey, traveling upward through the spine and activating the chakras as it rises. This journey typically spans several lifetimes, though it can be accelerated when guided by a highly evolved teacher. As spiritual progress is made, kundalini moves through the spine, energizing the chakras in new ways as they develop the ability to safely handle its power. Even in healthy individuals, the chakras often resemble delicate flowers, gently drooping, and holding only limited energy. With the assistance of mantra, kundalini strengthens the chakras, enhancing their capacity to store energy. This activation leads to better health, clearer perception of both this reality and others, and the attainment of spiritual powers.

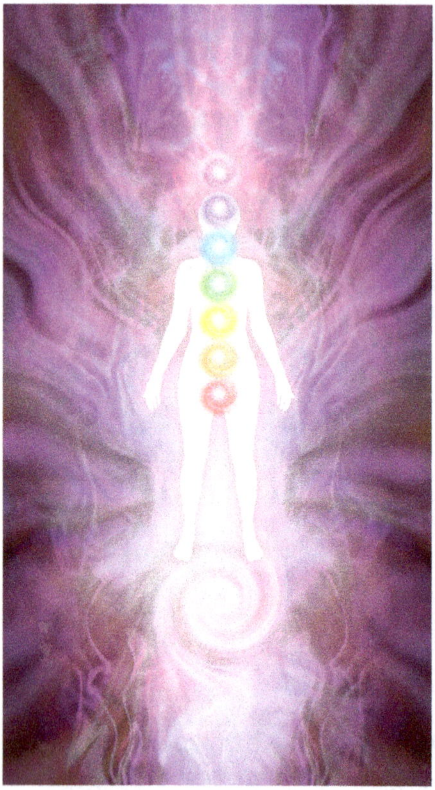

Kundalini is the supreme force driving our spiritual evolution. Mantra chanting expands the chakras' ability to hold spiritual energy and, as a result, they become prepared to receive the rising kundalini without causing harm to either the subtle or physical body. As kundalini rises through the spine, it energizes the chakras in transformative ways, sparking spiritual growth, deeper insight into our lives, and the emergence of esoteric abilities. Sometimes, this awakening can be triggered by powerful experiences such as listening to moving music, dancing, deeply connected or transcendent sexual encounters, or simply immersing oneself in nature. Walking on the beach, lying on the earth, or immersing in the ocean can all stir kundalini to awaken at new levels.

Some people have awakened kundalini as children, usually attributed to spiritual work they performed in previous lifetimes.

The esoteric gifts, *siddhis*, awakened as kundalini activates the chakras, include a range of heightened psychic and intuitive abilities. We will cover this in more depth in Chapter 4. These may manifest as:

◊ Enhanced psychic senses that expand perception beyond the physical realm.
◊ Mediumistic abilities, allowing communication with loved ones or others who have passed on.
◊ **Clairvoyance**, the ability to see future events or gain insight into hidden truths.
◊ **Clairaudience**, a mystical form of hearing through which one may receive messages from angels, ascended masters, or even the divine – conveying information about past or future events.
◊ **Claircognition**, a clear and immediate knowing – such as intuitively understanding what someone will say, or foreseeing outcomes without prior knowledge.
◊ **Clairsentience**, the ability to feel subtle energies within the body or sense what is happening energetically in oneself or others.

These abilities often unfold gradually as the chakras gain the capacity to hold and process the intensified energy of an awakened kundalini.

hindu deities

When we chant in Sanskrit, it invokes divine energetic forces that have been represented in the Vedic tradition as Hindu deities or principles. These principles existed as anthropomorphized energies before the Hindu religion and later became their gods and goddesses. One of the most commonly misunderstood aspects of Vedic teachings is the pantheon of gods and goddesses. Due to the presence of numerous deities, many people mistakenly assume that chanting in Sanskrit or following Vedic teachings, and later the religion of Hinduism, is polytheistic. This is not the case. Each god and goddess in Hinduism and Vedic teachings represents a specific principle of monotheistic divinity. Some believe these beings are liberated souls who have returned to guide humans on their spiritual journey, sometimes referred to in New Age terms as "Ascended Masters." Others see them as principles that have been anthropomorphized, making complex concepts more accessible and easier to understand. As Sri Muralidhar Pai likes to say, in the tradition of his father, Sadguru Sant Keshavadas, "Truth is one, but many are the names."

Most scholars and some mystics believe that the anthropomorphized Hindu deities are simply representations of energy. By giving them recognizable forms and personalities – complete with likes and dislikes – it becomes easier for everyone, including the illiterate, to relate to and understand the wide range of forces constantly influencing our lives. However, other mystics and sages view these deities as beings created long ago, some of whom were enlightened at the time of their creation. Others underwent spiritual practices to achieve enlightenment or realization. These beings then chose to assist humanity in its evolution, recognizing the potential of the species both individually and collectively.

the four aims

In the Vedic teachings, there are four aims of incarnation. Those aims are **Artha**, *Kama*, *Dharma*, and **Moksha**. *Artha* relates to worldly gains and other fruits we are here to experience on the earth plane during this incarnation. Why did we incarnate in a body anyway? The second aim is *Kama*, which means love or desire. The third aim is *Dharma*, basically our soul's purpose. What is my soul purpose? What is my *Dharma*? What are our gifts? What are our talents, and how can we share them? *Dharma* doesn't necessarily mean your job or your professional calling. The fourth aim of life or incarnation in a body, according to the Vedic teachings, is *Moksha*, which means liberation. Once you have obtained the three aims of *Artha*, *Kama*, and *Dharma*, it's time to release it all and seek *Moksha*.

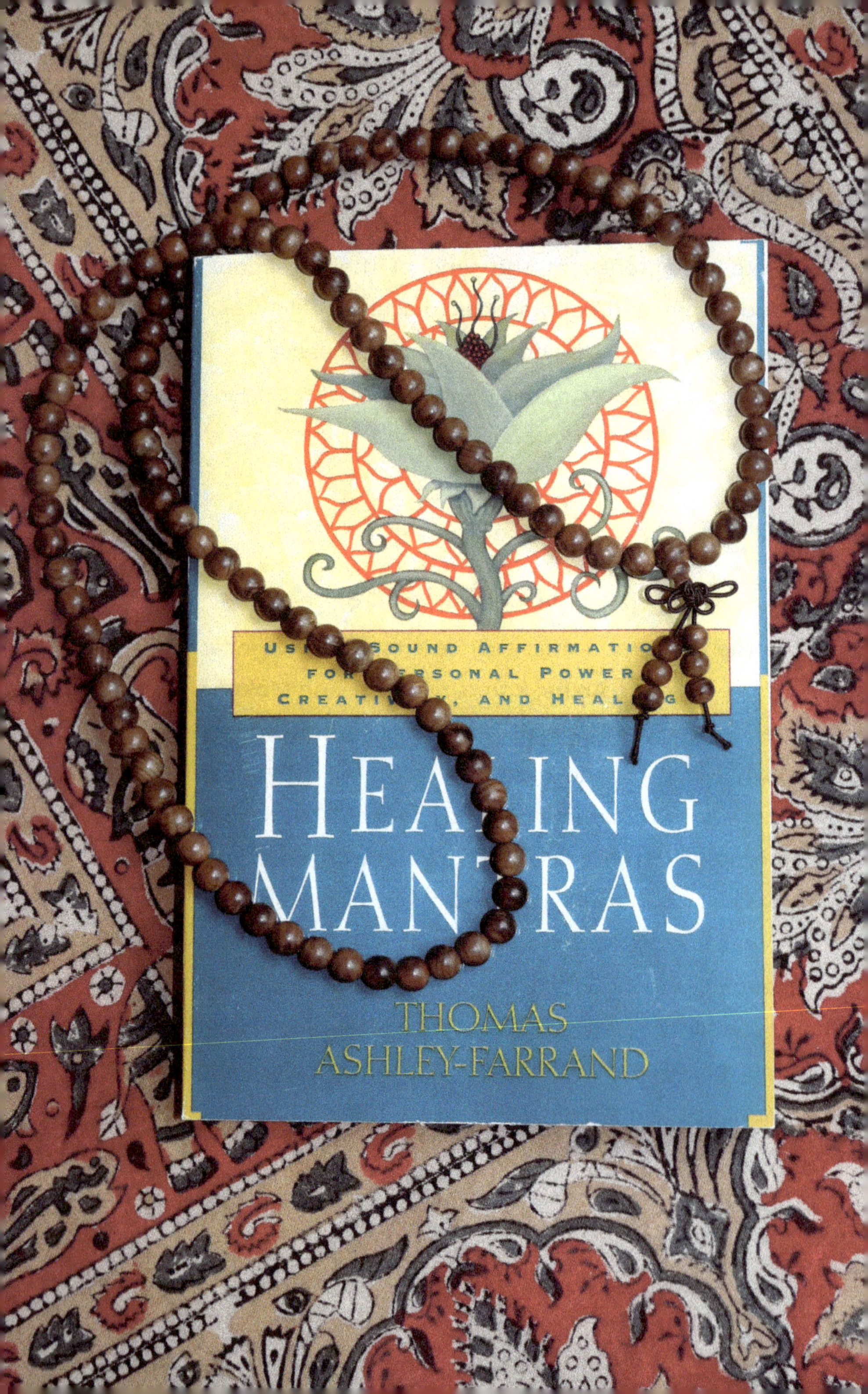
THOMAS
ASHLEY-FARRAND

"Mantras are energy-based sounds.
Mantras are also chakra-based sounds.
Mantra – combined with intention –
increases physical and spiritual benefits.
Mantras have only an approximate
language-based translation.
Mantra energizes prana.
Mantras are energy that
can be likened to fire."

~ Thomas Ashley-Farrand
Healing Mantras, p. 50

Seed Mantras

In Sanskrit mantra practice, the simplest and most potent sounds are known as *bija* mantras, or seed sounds. These are short, powerful syllables that channel energy in a precise and concentrated way. Their essence is so deeply rooted in pure vibration and energy that any attempt to translate them falls short. It would be like trying to translate putting one's finger in an electrical socket. Namadeva once described a seed mantra as an acorn containing the full potential of a mighty tree, whereas the full mantra is the tree itself, complete with branches and leaves. For example, the seed mantra "Shrim" encapsulates the energy of Lakshmi, and serves as the essence of the longer mantra "Om Shrim Maha Lakshmiyei Namaha." In other words, you can fast track your way to prosperity by simply chanting "Shrim."

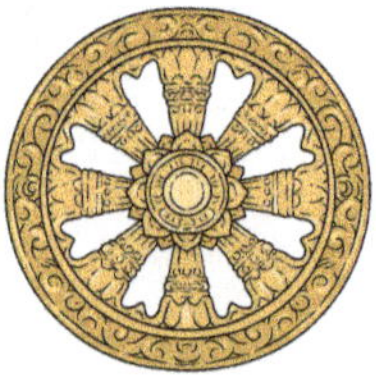

Om

Pronunciation: Om (also spelled Aum)
Bija for Universal Consciousness
Om is one of the most sacred and powerful mantras in Hinduism, Buddhism, Jainism, and various spiritual traditions. It is considered a primordial sound, believed to be the original vibration of the universe from which all creation emerged. Om symbolizes the totality of existence: creation, preservation, dissolution, and the transcendent.

gum

Pronunciation: Gum (as in chewing gum)

Bija for Ganesha

This seed sound calls in the **Ganesha/Ganapati** principle which removes obstacles and blockages. It is a good mantra for those who want to start chanting mantras. It can be used when initiating something new like a job, marriage, a new year, or moving into a new home.

shrim

Pronunciation: Shreem (rhymes with “stream”)

Bija for Lakshmi

This seed sound calls in the principle of prosperity, abundance, and divine feminine beauty, invoking the goddess Lakshmi. This is the sound for the principle of abundance. Abundance can come in the form of health, wealth, family and children, inner peace, friends, and healthy food to eat. This seed mantra is effective at bringing in money and resources when chanted 125,000 times (or 108 times). If one is guided to help others become more prosperous, especially when working with clients or students who need a financial boost, this mantra will work quickly. It’s also helpful to chant when you need help from other people for any reason.

aim

Pronunciation: I’m (rhymes with “time”)

Bija for **Saraswati**

This seed sound invokes the energy of Saraswati – wisdom, creativity, and eloquence. This is the seed sound ruling artistic and scientific endeavors as well as music and education. It invokes the principle of divine speech and gives words their power, including energizing Sanskrit mantras.

klim

Pronunciation: Kleem (rhymes with "dream")

Bija for attraction which can be used with deities such as Krishna, Lakshmi, or **Kali**

This seed sound invokes attraction. This is the seed for the principle of attraction. It can be chanted alone. This sound is commonly combined with other mantras to attract the object of desire. Because the power to attract things is so powerful, this seed is called Kama Bija or Desire Seed. *Kama* is Sanskrit for love and desire, as in the Kama Sutra. Remember never chant for a specific person, as this creates bad karma. Examples of "klim" added to other mantras are "Om Klim Krishnaya Namaha," for love. "Om Shrim Klim Maha Lakshmiyei Namaha," for prosperity. "Om Klim Kalikayei Namaha," for protection and power.

dum

Pronunciation: Doom

Bija for the principle of protection

This is personified as Goddess Durga, which invokes strength, and the divine feminine power. It is a *shakti* mantra, carrying the power of protection, destruction of negativity, and courage. A translation could be: "I invoke the protective, fiery, and transformative power of Durga."

krim

Pronunciation: Kreem

Bija for Goddess Kali and the energy of transformation, purification, and spiritual awakening.

This mantra is chanted for spiritual transformation, or to remove negative energies or attachments, to awaken inner strength and truth. It is often chanted in Tantric and Kundalini Yoga practices. It invokes "the force that destroys illusion and awakens spiritual truth."

hrim

Pronunciation: Hreem

Bija for the **Hrit Padma**, also known as "Sacred Heart"

If one practices this seed mantra with deep devotion and intensity, the true nature of the universe will be revealed to the seeker, just as it is. This is a seed sound for seeing through the illusion of this reality. It is found in both Vedic and Tibetan Buddhist practices. Chanting this seed mantra can also help one get in touch with their heart chakra and bring healing to the emotional heart. Vibrations of heat or buzzing in the heart, spine, and crown area have been reported by chanters of this mantra. People have also experienced emotional release such as unexpected crying or joy, or feelings of bliss and peace. The Hrit Padma is known by many names – Self, soul, **atman**, *jiva*, among others. It is the inner flame, the immortal essence within us that remains untouched and pure, carrying on through lifetimes until it ultimately reunites with the Divine. Esoteric traditions often describe it as the threefold flame. In classical Vedic practice, it is seen as a spark of **Narayana** – the source from which the entire cosmos emerges.

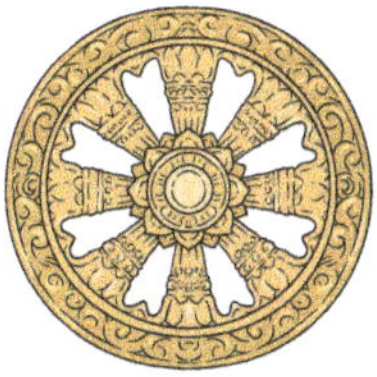

Namadeva advised to only use "Krim" under the supervision of a Sanskrit mantra teacher, and he suggested the "Klim" seed to be used with Kali as in "Om Klim Kalikayei Namaha."

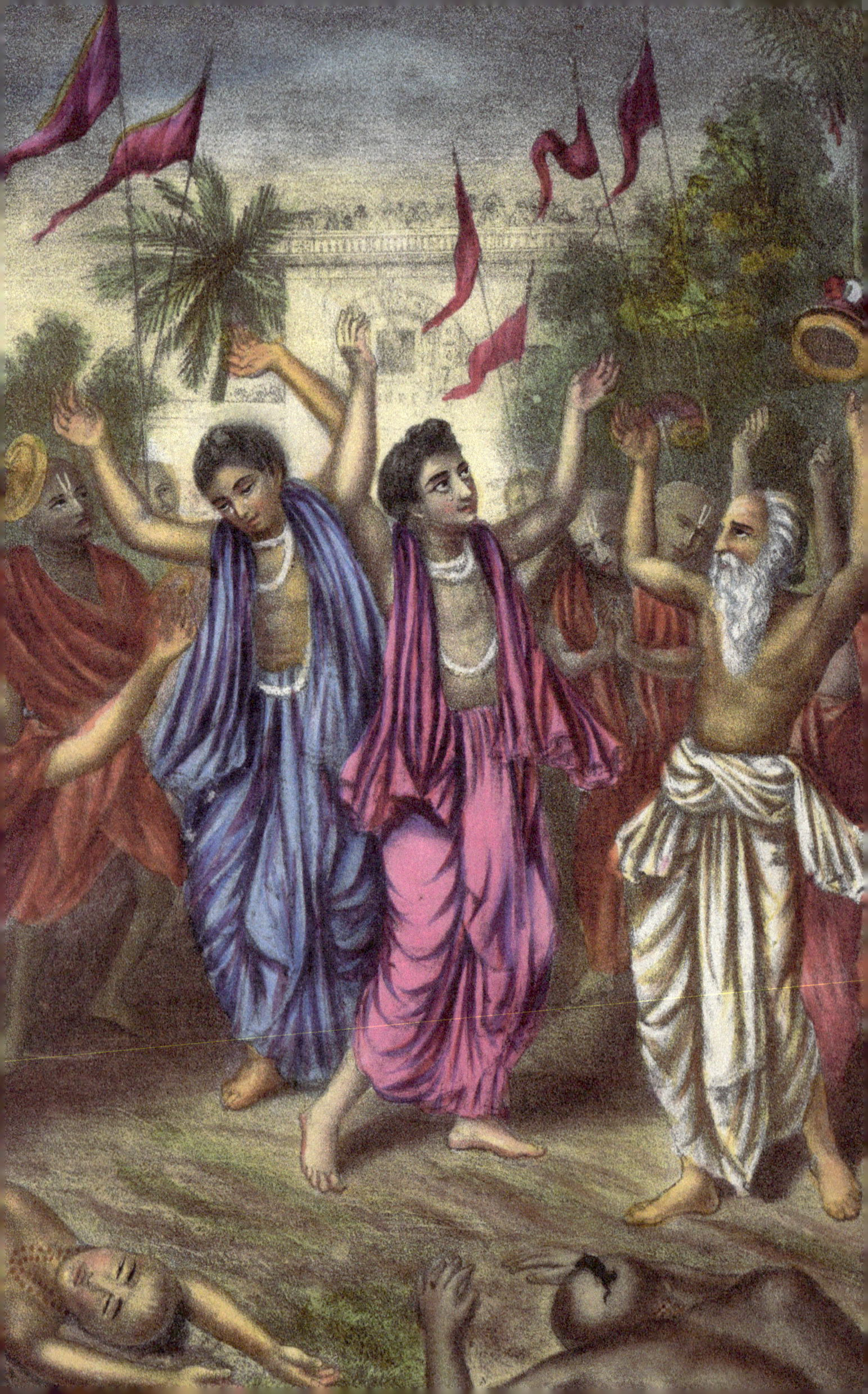

5
Chanting

Chanting in Sanskrit is an ancient Vedic practice, sometimes referred to as the Yoga of Sound. Sanskrit mantras are sacred sound formulas that shift our spiritual physiology. They clear blockages, both internally and externally, allowing us to be more receptive to our highest good. By removing obstacles, known or unknown in our body, mind, and energetic fields, Sanskrit mantras change our frequency so we become more magnetic to our soul powers and spiritual fruits.

As noted earlier, the literal meaning of mantra is to "free the mind." Chanting mantra is a method that can free us from our ingrained mental patterns and break the chains of any preordained life situations.

Sanskrit is known as **Deva Lingua**, the language of the gods, or the mother of tongues. It was linguists who described Sanskrit as such because it provides a root for many languages. Sanskrit is primarily an energy-based language, with meaning coming second. Sanskrit is fundamentally rooted in the concept of energy, with each letter and word carrying and invoking a distinct spiritual energy frequency. It really is a vibrational language. Until recently in history, approximately the past 70-100 years, it was only spoken by those *Brahmins* and priests in India who were initiated into these sacred sound formulas. It has come to the West with Gurus bringing this wisdom, beginning with Paramahamsa Yogananda and Swami Vivekananda, over 100 years ago. In the 1960s and 1970s a wave of Gurus came to the West, such as Yogi Bhajan, who introduced Kundalini Yoga, and Swami Muktananda, who introduced *shaktipat*. Many other gurus came during this time of awakening, including the lineage holder of these mantra teachings, Sadguru Sant Keshavadas and his wife, Guru Rama Mata. Namadeva learned Sanskrit mantras from them in the early 1970s.

The Sanskrit language is a tool for working with the subtle energy potential, represented by each of the hundreds of chakras within the energetic body. We have an energetic body in our spiritual physiology, which is referred to in yogic and Vedic teachings. The closest thing that most people relate to is the meridian system of energy in Chinese Medicine. In Acupuncture theory and practice, there are 12 meridians or channels that you cannot see on an X-ray but still can affect the movement of energy, health, and well-being in the physical body when activated by needles or touch. In the Vedic spiritual physiology there are seven main energy centers known as chakras and 72,000 *nadis* that can be opened and cleared when we chant in Sanskrit. Chanting in Sanskrit removes blockages in these subtle channels and removes *samskaras*, soul scars which show up as predispositions in this lifetime such as anxieties, fears, or addictions.

When we chant Sanskrit mantras we change our brainwaves and alter the templates of the mind which may be rooted in anxiety, trauma response, or repetitive thoughtforms that keep one cycling in a mental loop. Mantras can clear old patterns such as debilitating anxiety, worry, or fear. Mantras circumvent and rewire mental and psychological default tendencies. There are many benefits from mitigating repeating mental patterns that keep us cycling in fear, anxiety, or stressful thoughts. A spiritual teacher from the 1970s once said that the rewiring of brain patterning is like a cassette tape that keeps rewinding in the mind. Mantra breaks that tape and upgrades your mental program. Making the analogy in current terms we could say that mantra offers new internal software which optimizes your psychoneurological interface. When the mind is calmed, we can attract more positive manifestations into our lives. Chanting in Sanskrit brings resonance to the attainment that one is chanting for, such as health or wealth. For instance, if someone is chanting mantras to Lakshmi, the Goddess of prosperity and abundance, their pre-existing thought patterns of scarcity and lack can become subdued and mitigated, whether they are aware of these limiting beliefs or they are buried deep in the subconscious. Calming the mind and senses, and quelling old patterns won't happen overnight, but chanting mantras can chip away at the mental clutter and karmic repercussions.

When one chants mantras, it creates a vibrational upliftment that promotes mental clarity and calmness. While the primary effects are mental and energetic, chanting can also support physical relaxation. Mantras work on the *nadis* – the body's "superhighways" – and when these channels are open, they help the body release tension, clear the bronchial passages, and achieve a state of deep relaxation. Additionally, chanting activates the chakras, which helps regulate and organize the glandular system, supporting higher bodily functions and, in some cases, enabling the attainment of *siddhis*.

Chanting mantras can help heal and recalibrate the nervous system, effectively offering a reset. When the body's energy channels are opened through sound, they influence the brain's circuitry, especially in individuals whose systems are overstimulated due to stress, anxiety, or trauma. Mantras help break up old neurological patterns and support the creation of new neural pathways. They open subtle portals within the nervous system where trauma is often stored, allowing these imprints to be released and integrated.

As discussed in relation to the chakras, the seven main energy centers correspond to the body's glandular system. When mantras are chanted, they stimulate the endocrine glands, activating and balancing their functions. This activation promotes a state of relaxation by influencing brainwave activity, helping to interrupt patterns of fight-or-flight response. In effect, mantra chanting can short-circuit stress responses, allowing the body's systems to recalibrate. This aligns with scientific research on the relaxation response, which shows how intentional practices like chanting can bring the body and mind into a state of deep rest and renewal.

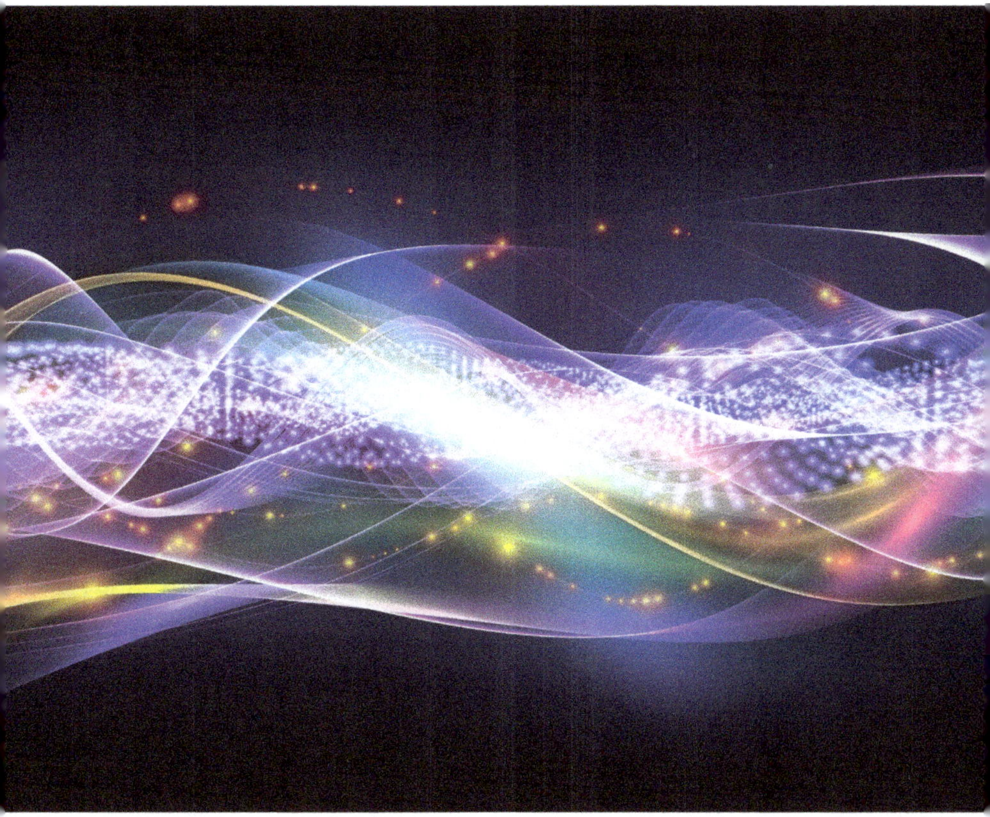

how to chant

Dr. Alexi Jardine Martel

When chanting mantras, it is tradition to say them on a **mala**, a necklace made of 108 round crystals, seeds, or beads plus an additional foundational one known as the *meru* bead which hangs lower than the rest. The spiritual practitioner holds the first bead (one next to the *meru* bead, but not the *meru* bead itself) in their hand between their thumb and middle finger and begins the mantra **japa** (the practice of chanting on a mala) by saying the mantra one time while holding the bead. Then they use their thumb to advance to the next bead, moving away from the *meru* bead, and say the mantra again, repeating the process of saying the mantra once for each bead until they reach the *meru* bead. By this point, they will have said 108 repetitions of the mantra. This is one mala. 108 is a sacred number in the Vedic tradition for a number of reasons, so it is also the standard measurement of a single *japa* session reciting the mantra. One is welcome to chant more than one mala's worth of mantras in a single setting. If you wish to continue after completing one mala, you then repeat the process but move the beads in the opposite direction by pulling them towards you. In this way you avoid crossing over the *meru* bead, which is never chanted on itself.

One can practice mantra *japa* in this way by reciting the mantra out loud, by whispering it, or even by saying it silently. Different spiritual authorities debate which method is best, but a common consensus is that vocally saying the mantra out loud directly impacts your body and physical environment, while saying it silently focuses the effects on the mind. Personally, I prefer to say mantras out loud as I feel it benefits all aspects of my being. This is especially useful when working with mantras with the intention of healing or increasing physical vitality (*prana*), as the physical vibration of the spoken mantra permeates your physical body directly this way. However, as always with mantras, intention and attention are key determinants in the efficacy of chanting. If you find that your mind wanders while reciting the mantra out loud but you can focus on it better when you say it silently then that might be the ideal approach for you. The same rule applies to choosing a mantra to chant as choosing how you chant it – the best approach for you is the one that you will (consistently) do.

Attention is a key ingredient to a successful mantra practice, as we have already discussed. The role of intention is also worth highlighting. Typically one embarks on a mantra practice to affect some positive change within one's life, and with that comes an intended goal or intention for the practice. It is perfectly fine to say a mantra casually if it resonates with you intuitively and you want to explore its energy to see what happens. However, if you want to apply mantras as spiritual levers to improve some part of your life – such as health, wealth, relationships, connection to the Divine – then a focused practice or mantra discipline is the recommended approach. A typical minimum mantra discipline to make a lasting change in your life is the 40-day discipline. As the name implies, this involves chanting the mantra for 40 days in a row without missing a day. The amount you chant per day can vary based on your available time and desired intensity, but a common minimum amount is at least one mala, or 108 repetitions of the mantra per day. The more you say, the more you benefit, but one mala per day for 40 days will make a meaningful impact on your spiritual physiology and your karma. If you miss a day within the 40-day discipline, it does mean that you would need to start over again. However, do not be discouraged if this happens to you because the mantras that you previously chanted are not wasted. As Lord **Krishna**, an **avatar** of God, according to Vedic text the Bhagavad Gita, said, "On this path no effort ever goes to waste and there is no failure. Even a little practice of this will protect you from the cycle of death and rebirth."*

What's in a Day?

When embarking on a 40-day discipline of mantra *japa* following the Vedic spiritual tradition, it's worth noting what exactly marks a day in the tradition. In the Vedic reckoning,

* Jack Hawley, *The Bhagavad Gita: A Walkthrough for Westerners* (New World Library, 2011), 19.

a day begins at sunrise and does not end until the following sunrise, which marks the start of the next day. So, there is no requirement to complete your mantra practice exclusively when the sun is up or even before midnight on a given calendar day. However, if the sun rises on a new day without you having completed your mantra practice the previous day or if you go to sleep for the night and fall asleep before chanting, this does end the 40-day practice.

Alternatives to Mala Japa

Sometimes people prefer to chant without the use of a mala. This is fine. You can set aside five or ten minutes to focus on chanting or you can chant as you drive, as you do chores, or when you go for a walk. If you want to chant while in public spaces, it's recommended to do so silently so as not to alarm strangers. The more you chant, the more powerful the mantra's effects will be, so it really is a case of the more the merrier. It can be fun and gratifying to use a stopwatch on a clock app on your phone to record how long you chanted. If you are interested in a 40-day discipline but don't want to use a mala, it's a good idea to find out how long it takes you to say 108 repetitions of the mantra and set aside that amount of time for focused chanting each day of your discipline. For most mantras included in this book it takes about five minutes to say 108 repetitions.

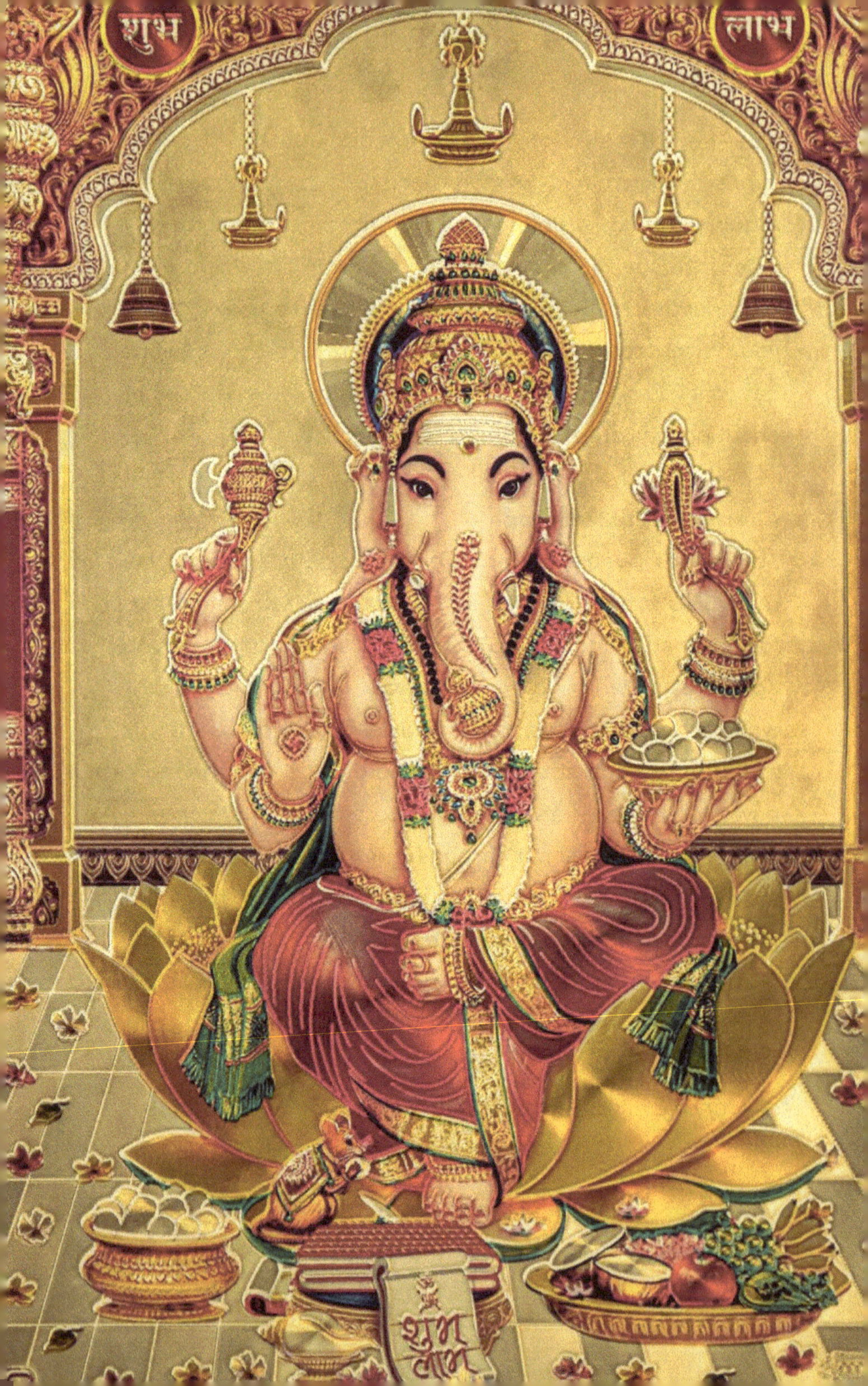
शुभ
लाभ
शुभ लाभ

3
Mantras to Remove Obstacles

The Ganesha Principle

Who is Ganesha and why does he have an elephant head? Known as Ganapathi and Ganesha, he is the elephant-headed god revered by Hindus. According to legend, he was created by his mother, **Parvati**, during a time of loneliness while her husband, Shiva, the Divine Masculine, was away for long periods of time. As the embodiment of the Divine Mother and the very power of the universe, Parvati desired a companion and protector. To fulfill this need, she created a handsome boy. One day, as she went to take a bath she told Ganesha to stand guard and prevent any intruders from entering. While she was bathing, Shiva returned home, anxious to see his beloved wife, but an impetuous 12-year-old boy stopped him and demanded he halt. Shiva was taken by the handsome lad, but then proceeded to enter the house. Ganesha refused to let Shiva enter, and Shiva became quite perturbed, asking this young upstart if he knew who he was messing with. Ganesha, not knowing this was his father or his universal status and power, responded by saying he didn't care who he was but he couldn't enter the home. Shiva became so enraged he sent an angry glance from his third eye to the boy, which cut off his head and it fell to the ground. Parvati rushed out of the bath, transforming into the wrathful Kali, raging at Shiva. The Lord of all realms was no match for his angry wife. Shiva explained he did not know who the boy was but realized he was so devoted to Parvati, that he stood up against him, the powerful god Shiva. The solution was that Shiva would find a way to bring him back to life, by finding a new head from the first creature he encounters who had just died. Shiva and Parvati then walked through the divine countryside together and saw a young elephant who had just died. Shiva grabbed the head of the elephant and placed it on the body of Parvati's son, Ganesha. He sprang to life as the beautiful boy with an elephant head, ever to be known as Ganesha. Thus the Ganesha/Ganapathi principle was born, with the ability to remove obstacles and so much more. Shiva bestowed the big elephant headed boy with divine wisdom, *buddhi*, and divine power, *siddhi*. According to Sadguru Sant Keshavadas: "*Buddhi* is that illumined intellect whereby your mind is so alert that in your work you are able to see everything by the power of that illumination. And *siddhi* is the attainment not only of supernatural powers but also of spiritual fulfillment."*

* Sadguru Sant Keshavadas, *Lord Ganesha* (Vishwa Dharma Publications, 1988), 6.

ganesha

Ganesha is perhaps the most widely recognized Vedic deity in the Western World, as the contemporary yoga culture has embraced him fully. Ganesha's presence is evident in many yoga studios with his image adorning walls, yoga apparel, and even his statues holding court in the front of the room with the yoga teacher. Many yoga students and teachers are minimally informed about what Ganesha symbolizes beyond knowing he is the remover of obstacles. Traditionally, in India, Ganesha is invoked at the beginning of an event or endeavor, such as starting a business or new job, getting married, moving into a new home, blessing a baby, or embarking on any new venture to ensure auspicious results. The Ganesha principle in Vedic teachings holds great importance, as this is the deity perpetually honored at the beginning of anything new, including a ceremony, **sadhana** (spiritual practice), or mantra discipline. When one is embarking on the path of chanting Sanskrit, Ganesha mantras are the first ones to embrace. Ganesha is always invoked at the beginning of any endeavor, spiritual practice, job, or other fresh start to receive the blessings of Ganesha by removing obstacles to a successful undertaking.

why ganesha is honored first: the story of the celestial race

According to one of the most well-known stories, the practice of chanting Ganesha first comes from an incident involving the gods Shiva and **Vishnu** during a great dispute. The celestials held a great competition to determine which among them should be honored first in all rituals. The challenge was simple in theory but daunting in execution: whoever could circle the universe three times and return first would be granted this honor. The celestials immediately took off on their powerful mounts – swift birds, majestic lions, and magical beasts. But Ganesha, with the head of an elephant and a round, heavy body, rode a small rat, the slowest of all vehicles. He paused, not out of hesitation, but out of deep thought.

Ganesha calmly considered the situation:

- All the deities desired to be honored first.
- The race was a test – not just of speed, but of insight.
- The goal was to circle the entire universe three times.
- His own mount, a humble rat, made a literal race unwinnable.
- Most importantly, the race had been devised by his parents, Shiva and Parvati – divine embodiments of cosmic power and love – who would not be racing but presiding over the event.

Somewhere in these details lay the answer. Ganesha began to move slowly toward his mother, Parvati, still contemplating the true nature of the challenge. When he was just a few steps away, she turned and smiled at him with radiant affection. In that moment, the solution illuminated his mind.

Without pause, Ganesha mounted his rat and began riding in a circle around his mother. He completed three full revolutions, his focus unwavering. As he finished, Shiva approached, placed a golden crown upon Ganesha's head, and declared him the winner.

When the other deities returned, panting and surprised to see Ganesha already crowned, some were confused, even irritated. Shiva invited Ganesha to explain. Ganesha spoke calmly and clearly:

> *To me, the universe is not just stars and space. My Divine Mother embodies the entire cosmos. By circling her three times, I have honored the full breadth of creation – with heart, mind, and intention. She is the origin of all, and by moving around her, I have traveled the universe itself. My Mother is the entire world.*

Then he gently asked, *Who among you can say I am wrong?* The gods fell silent, awed by his insight and devotion. One by one, they bowed their heads in respect. A great cheer arose: **"Salutations to Ganesha! Salutations to Parvati – Divine Mother and body of the Cosmos!"**

From that day forward, it was established that Ganesha would be honored first – in every ritual, every sacred ceremony, and every new beginning – as a symbol of wisdom, devotion, and right understanding.

When one chants Ganesha mantras they can activate the energy of *siddhi,* or magical displays in their life. There is something known as **mantra siddhi**, which means that when we have chanted a specific mantra a certain number of times, usually 250,000+ repetitions, depending on our individual karma, that mantra will remarkably yield its fruit in our life. For instance, the Ganesha foundation *(mula)* mantra is "Om Gum Ganapatayei Namaha," and I have experienced the results of mantra *siddhi* with that mantra in a specific way.

Chanting Ganesha mantras will give power combined with wisdom. Ganesha blesses the chanter with *buddhi* and *siddhi*. Power combined with wisdom can make a heaven on earth.

Ganesha is the energy we chant for when we want to remove obstacles or blockages. This includes astrological challenges that arise when we're unsure which planets in our chart may be causing difficulties – whether due to their natal positions or current transits. It's particularly relevant for those who aren't astrologers or don't yet know their natal chart, but sense that a planet is under stress. But since the deity Ganesha holds the whole cosmos in his belly, we can chant to him for any astrological issue as well.

om gum ganapatayei namaha

Om Gum Guh-nuh-puh-tuh-yei Nahm-ah-ha

Om – Primordial sound, universal consciousness
Gum – *Bija* sound of Ganesha
Ganapatayei – To Ganesha (Lord of the *ganas,* celestial attendants)
Namaha – I bow , salutations

Salutations to Lord Ganesha, remover of obstacles and lord of the multitudes.

The Ganapati Mantra is used for removing obstacles. It bestows blessings when embarking upon a new endeavor, job, or career, and before entering into a contract or business. This crowns the outcome of these new initiatives with success. In the Vedic teachings the remover of obstacles is the Ganapathi principle. *Gana* means power in Sanskrit and *pathi* means spouse. So the literal translation of Ganapathi is the spouse of power. Ganapathi is a name for the Vedic deity or principle of Ganesha, who is a manifestation of the divine principle. *Gana-Esha* translates to "Ruler of power."

This *mula* mantra of Ganesha is used to usher in auspicious outcomes to a new project or undertaking. This mantra removes obstacles or blocks, known or unknown, in our body, mind, and spirit. This includes obstacles coming from outside ourselves, including from other people or circumstances.

This is the most widely prescribed mantra I have given to clients and students over the years as a Sanskrit mantra instructor. They have shared stories of this mantra helping them with situations that felt overwhelming or insurmountable and after chanting the mantra, issues were mitigated, and solutions appeared. Problems were cleared. This is usually the first mantra I will recommend to clients, especially those who are new to mantra. They embrace chanting it and usually see a shift in their circumstances within 48 hours. Once the pronunciation is down, it becomes very natural to chant. Most people take to it easily – and even kids love it.

Clients have told me they chant it when traveling to make things go smoothly. One of my mantra students shared the story of flying on a puddle jumper plane and hitting intense turbulence, so she immediately grabbed her mala and started chanting "Om Gum Ganapatayei Namaha," and in no time the turbulence disappeared and they arrived at their destination intact. I have also used this mantra for traveling, to make connections on time, for smooth flying, and sometimes the planes will arrive early!

As I've shared, I've experienced what is known as *mantra siddhi* – the awakening of a mantra's full potency – through chanting "Om Gum Ganapatayei Namaha." The moment I begin to chant, its effects begin to ripple through the seen and unseen. One particular area where this has revealed itself consistently is while driving. On numerous occasions, when I've found myself stuck behind slow-moving traffic, I'll begin chanting – and within minutes, the path ahead opens. Cars shift, lanes clear, and I'm free to move forward.

I don't invoke this mantra frivolously. But when I'm en route to teach, offer healing, or be of service, Ganesha – the great remover of obstacles – responds. There's a sacred intelligence at play, one that recognizes the intention behind the chant and clears the way not just on the road, but in the energetic field surrounding the moment.

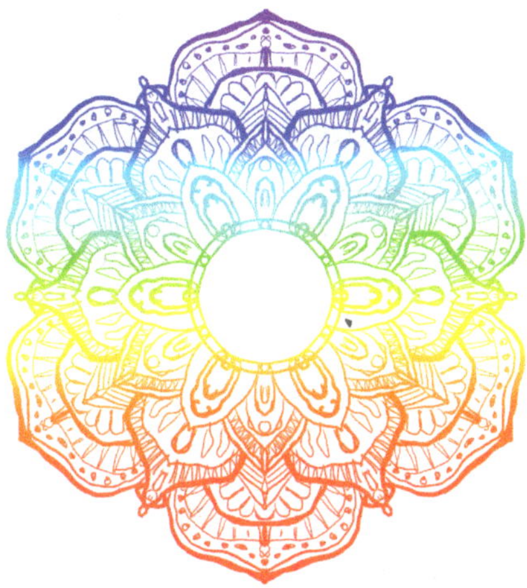

Om Lakshmi Ganapatayei Namaha

Om Laksh-mee Guh-nuh-puh-tuh-yei Nahm-ah-ha

Om – Primordial sound, universal consciousness
Lakshmi – Goddess of wealth, abundance
Ganapatayei – To Ganesha
Namaha – I bow , salutations

Salutations to Lakshmi-Ganapati, the aspect of Ganesha who brings wealth and prosperity.

This mantra invokes both the Ganapati principle and Lakshmi, goddess of abundance, to remove blocks to attracting greater abundance. It has the power of the foundational mantra of Ganesha combined with the principle of prosperity.

This mantra unites the energies of Lakshmi and Ganesha to remove obstacles blocking prosperity. Before chanting, meditate on the specific issue you wish to clear. It is also advised to meditate on the color gold or a golden Ganesha.

This mantra is extremely effective in removing subconscious blocks to receiving blessings of all types, including prosperity. It has helped my clients clear issues around self worth or lack consciousness. Lakshmi bestows access to more prosperity while Ganesha removes any obstacles whether they be internal or external. Sadguru Sant Keshavadas recommended that those who want wealth and prosperity to, "meditate on the golden-colored Ganesha and say this prayer."*

"Om Lakshmi Ganapatayei Namaha" is one of my favorite mantras to recommend to clients over the past 20+ years. My client Charles, an avid mantra chanter and Vedic Astrologer, swears by this mantra for bringing in quick cash. This is one of his experiences after chanting this mantra: "During a reading with Jill, I expressed concerns regarding financial difficulties and she recommended that I chant 'Om Lakshmi Ganapataye Namaha'... to make things 'more affordable.' I got in the habit of doing this when I was concerned about finances but I would also chant this mantra passively when I went shopping for necessities, groceries, etc. One day, I went shopping for new work shoes. I found a pair that fit my needs but I was concerned about the price. At the check out desk I was chanting this mantra in my head and asked the cashier if the store was offering any special discounts. After looking through a book of discounts she told me could offer me 25% off. This is just one of many examples of success with this mantra."

* Sadguru Sant Keshavadas, *Lord Ganesha* (Vishwa Dharma Publications, 1988), 28.

om kshipra prasadaya namaha

Om Kship-ra Pra-sa-da-ya Nahm-ah-ha

(KSHIH → like "kish" but with a soft "sh" blended into the "k" -pruh)

Om – Sacred sound
Kshipra – Quick, immediate
Prasadaya – Bestower of grace or blessings
Namaha – I bow

Salutations to the one who grants blessings swiftly.

This mantra is a prayer to Lord Ganesha, invoking his swift blessings and grace. *Kshipra* means instantaneous, so this mantra can deliver instant blessings. It can bring relief to remove some oppressive obstacle, or ease a situation which feels insurmountable, especially when combined with "Om Gum Ganapatayei Namaha." If one is faced with financial difficulties that need immediate attention, "Om Kshipra Prasadaya Namaha" can be combined with a Lakshmi mantra, such as "Shrim."

This mantra combination can ease the intensity of the pending financial concern and have a solution appear, sometimes in the form of unexpected money. It is also very protective when combined with "Om Dum Durgayei Namaha," to keep danger or unwieldy circumstances away. According to Sadguru Sant Keshavadas, "if some danger is coming your way and you don't know how to get rid of that trouble, with true devotion, practice this mantra for quick blessing."*

This mantra is one of the hidden gems in my toolbox – a "secret weapon" I sometimes forget to use but love sharing. It's especially powerful in a "mantra stack," a sequence of complementary mantras chanted together to amplify their effects.

I've seen remarkable results when clients use this mantra. One striking example is Carol, a photographer who came to me deeply anxious and behind on her mortgage. She was short $9,000 on a $10,000 payment due within days and had no upcoming work. For weeks, she had been chanting "Om Gum Ganapatayei Namaha" and "Om Shrim Maha Lakshmiyei Namaha" with dedication, but now she needed immediate help.

I suggested she add "Om Kshipra Prasadaya Namaha" to her practice and make it her main focus. Carol began repeating the mantra as she drove home from our session. During that drive, a former client called, urgently needing photos for a new business launch within days. Carol agreed and scheduled the shoot for the next day. That evening, the client confirmed and paid her $10,000 in advance. Within two hours of chanting "Om Kshipra Prasadaya Namaha," Carol had manifested exactly what she needed to save her home.

* Sadguru Sant Keshavadas, *Lord Ganesha* (Vishwa Dharma Publications, 1988), 32.

om sri siddhi vinayakaya namaha

Om Shree Sid-dhi Vi-na-ya-ka-ya Nahm-ah-ha

Om – Sacred sound
Sri – Reverence, auspiciousness
Siddhi – Spiritual power or success
Vinayakaya – To Vinayaka (another name for Ganesha)
Namaha – I bow

Salutations to the revered Vinayaka who grants success and accomplishments.

This mantra can also be translated as, "Om, may that Vinayaka (Ganapati/Ganesha principle) bestow upon me the state of perfection and the powers inherent in it." This mantra can help the aspirant attain the *siddhi* or special blessings of Ganesha. Some examples of *siddhis* were described earlier in the book such clairvoyance, clairaudience, prophecy, knowledge of one's past lives, knowledge of past, present and future, freedom from hunger and thirst, and freedom from the effects of heat and cold. According to Namadeva, this mantra "invokes energy, accelerating the process of inner perfection. As part of the process, supramundane abilities will manifest at some point. This mantra invokes the Grace of Ganesha during this Kali Yuga."*

* Thomas-Ashley Farrand, *Teacher of Mantra Instruction Manual* (Saraswati Publications, 2008) 209.

This mantra salutes and invokes the power of Ganesha to overcome evil and overcome any difficulty. It brings success in the wake of all activities. Vinayaka is the Lord of Problems, so they will start to resolve and come under control when chanting this mantra.

I chant this mantra sometimes before doing readings for clients, to obtain Ganesha's assistance in helping the session go well. I have noticed that after chanting this mantra, the *siddhis* of clairaudience and prophecy seem to flow forth more effortlessly during the reading.

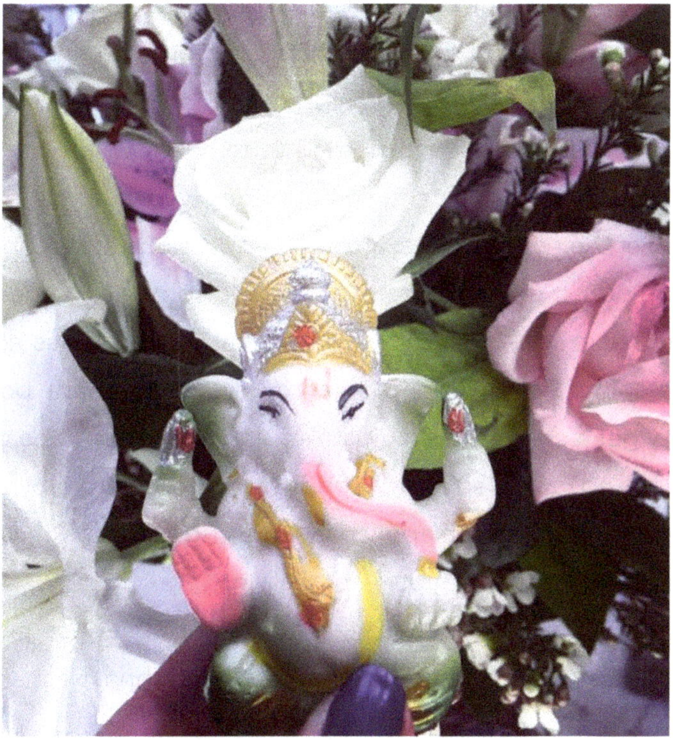

Om Vighna Nashanaya Namaha

Om Vig-na Na-sha-na-ya Nahm-ah-ha

Om – Sacred sound
Vighna – Obstacles
Nashanaya – Destroyer or remover
Namaha – I bow

Salutations to the remover of obstacles.

This mantra also translates to: "Salutations to Ganesha as the dissolver of blockages." It invokes Ganesha to remove every impediment in your life. By consistently chanting this mantra with devotion all obstacles and blocked energy are released.

This is a very good mantra to chant when you feel there are obstacles or forces opposing you but you're not sure of their origin. For example, are these obstacles coming from others or from circumstances or from within oneself? It is also a very good mantra for clearing blockages along the spine. I recommend it to my clients to chant before they get a chiropractic adjustment or other form of healing, to open up the spinal channel before their therapy. This mantra could also be applied as a healing mantra with other mantras from the chapter on healing.

I suggested to my chiropractor that just before he adjust clients that he chant "Om Vighna Nashanaya

Namaha" and notice if there was a difference or ease in his chiropractic adjustments. The answer was a resounding "Yes!" He felt as if his hands were being guided on the patient's back right to where they were blocked and energy was stuck. One patient was amazed at how he honed in on the place where they felt pain. There was also so much heat that was released after the stuck area was adjusted.

I have also used this mantra when I feel I need a chiropractic adjustment but can't get to the chiropractor for several days. Chanting this mantra opens up the spinal pathway and I can feel the blocked energy release and then clear up through the *nadis*.

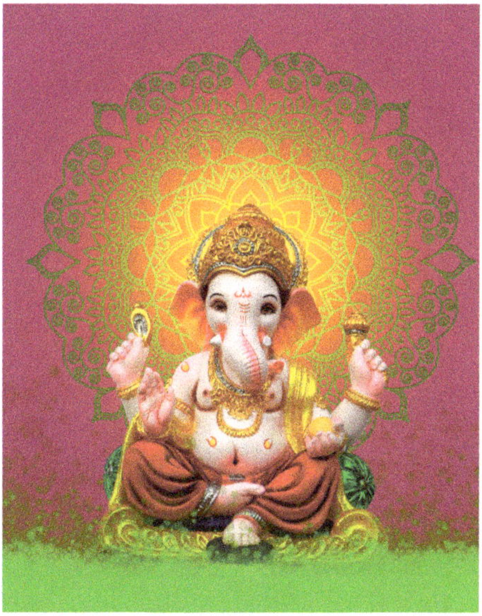

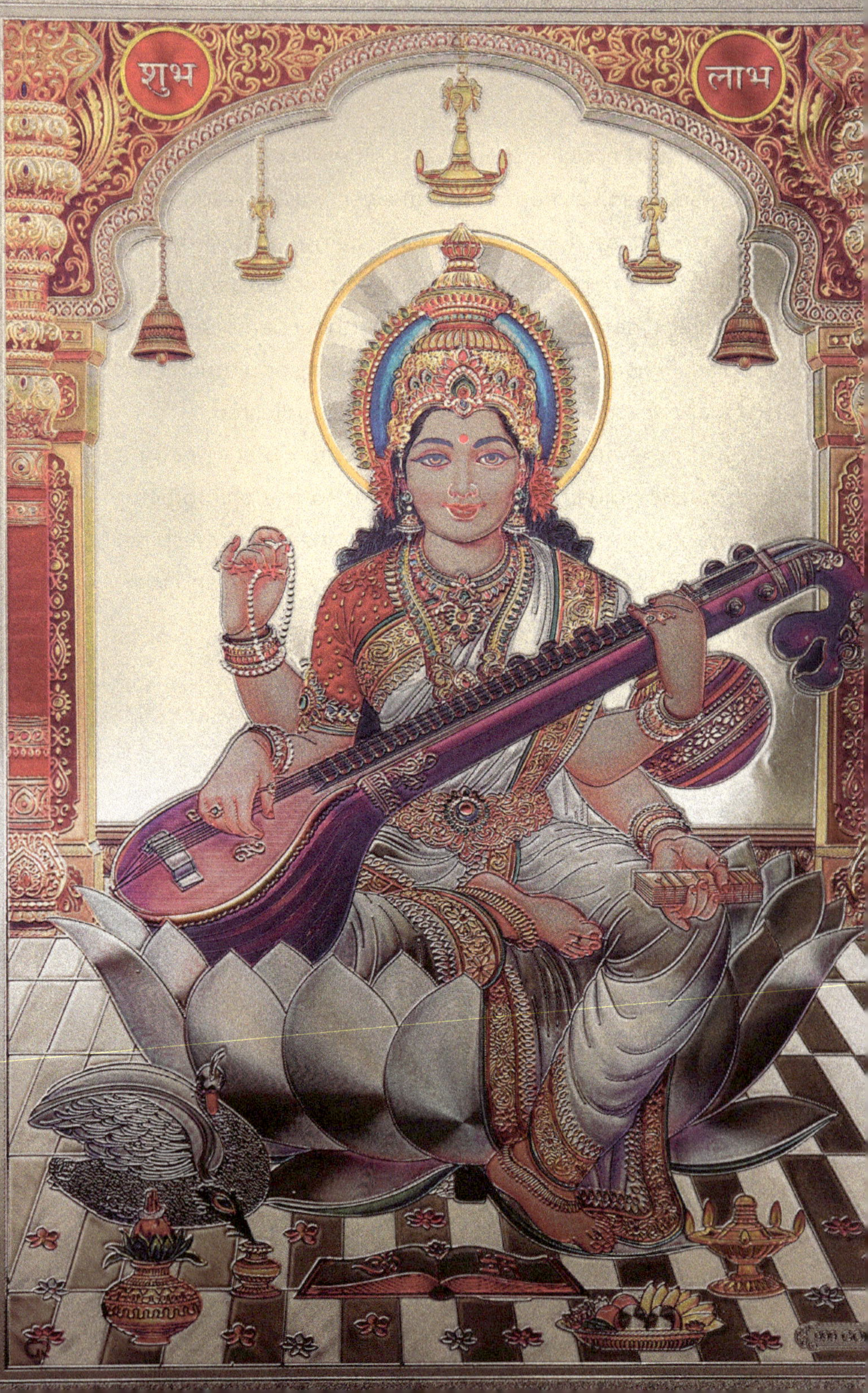
शुभ
लाभ

4
Mantras for Developing Intuition

The Saraswati Principle

Saraswati is often depicted holding a **vina** (a classical stringed instrument) in one hand and a mala (prayer beads) in the other, with a book resting at her feet. The mala symbolizes concentration, discipline, and spiritual practice. The *vina* represents harmony, music, and the rhythm of life. The book represents the *vedas* or scriptures, symbolizing sacred knowledge and learning. Saraswati's vehicle is a white **lotus** or swan symbolizing purity and discernment, separating truth from illusion. Saraswati wears white clothing denoting purity, simplicity, and transcendence.

She embodies the feminine force that awakens, sustains, and refines artistic, academic, and spiritual pursuits. Mothers in India frequently chant Saraswati mantras on behalf of their children to support their success in education and learning.

Among the divine feminine archetypes, Saraswati is the least known in the West. While goddesses like Lakshmi (abundance), Durga (protection), and Kali (transformation and ego dissolution) are more widely recognized, Saraswati remains quietly revered.

This may be because Saraswati is the *shakti* of true wisdom – the gateway to pure spiritual knowledge, discernment, and subtle perception. In many Eastern traditions, such knowledge has historically been kept esoteric and protected, passed only to those prepared to receive it. Saraswati represents that hidden current – the subtle, refined intelligence that guides us beyond information and into realization.

She embodies the divine feminine principle of wisdom, learning, speech, creativity, and spiritual insight. Her name comes from the Sanskrit root *saras* meaning flow and *vati* meaning "she who has" – indicating a flowing, dynamic current of consciousness, often associated with language, thought, and intuition.

Saraswati activates the power of divine speech and offers creative inspiration for poets, musicians, teachers, and seekers of high truth. She is **Jnana** *shakti*, the power of knowledge and insight and helps with the development of intuition and connection to the higher mind. She is the consort of Brahma, the Creator, suggesting that knowledge and wisdom are necessary for creation to unfold.

Devotees invoke Saraswati for academic success, artistic and musical inspiration and expression, spiritual clarity, and eloquence in speech.

According to Thomas Ashley-Farrand, "At a deeper level, Saraswati principle governs the development and manifestation of spiritual knowledge. Many Himalayan teachers adopt 'Saraswati' as part of their spiritual name, which is the vibration of wisdom and knowledge as power."*

Intuition

It seems these days increasing numbers of people are seeking to become more intuitive. That's a good thing! It's an empowering experience to tune into your higher mind and discern the truth for yourself, instead of relying on internet psychics and soothsayers. People have sought me out as a professional astrologer, psychic, and healer for over 30 years, with the burning questions: "How can I become more intuitive?" "What did you do to become intuitive and be able to give such accurate psychic readings over the years?"

My answer to those questions is that I developed psychic gifts that showed up in my youth. In retrospect, these skills are probably a *siddhi* or talent I cultivated in a previous life by performing yogic practices and spiritual devotion. I have also worked hard as an adult to develop my gifts through practice and application of various metaphysical techniques, including Sanskrit mantras. However, as a kid and teenager, I pursued a much more academic route, and it was when I discovered astrology and the Tarot at 15 that I realized it felt familiar and I had some

* Thomas Ashley-Farrand, *Teacher of Mantra Instruction Manual* (Saraswati Publications, 2008), 196.

natural gifts in giving readings. It wasn't necessarily an asset during my youth, as I was focused on the pursuit of education. I couldn't really expand upon it until after my undergraduate years in college, and then ultimately earned a Masters Degree in Counseling Psychology to legitimize my esoteric endeavors. During the era I grew up in the psychic world and astrology was viewed as fringe and even witchy, unlike the current times where the internet has exploded these subjects into the mainstream. I also cultivated my talents by doing psychic and astrology readings for people (initially for free), researching as much as I could find on the mystical world, practicing and teaching yoga (before it became mainstream), and following the Vedic path of teachings on consciousness and mantra. I feel yogic practices are key in developing the *siddhis*. Yoga was traditionally a science that helped the practitioner or yogi develop their full human potential and beyond.

The important point that I tell people when they ask me how they can become more intuitive, is that it is a natural human skill, and we all have these abilities whether latent, developing, or blossoming. I do believe that even if one has innate intuitive wisdom that is accurate, it must be consistently cultivated by doing certain practices. As the saying goes, "if you don't use it, you lose it."

It is crucial now more than ever to be able to discern the truth for oneself. Truth is a scarce commodity these days and everyone is spouting their version of it through political platforms, media, alternative media outlets, and social media. And it has been proven that these sources are all manipulated in one way or another. It is very confusing for many to decipher what is real and what is a narrative, and they can be led astray down a rabbit hole of misperceptions and falsehoods.

But what if there was a way to *know* the truth for yourself? The path isn't through one's ego or subconscious but by tuning into the wisdom of the soul, which is connected to divine wisdom. The ego and subconscious must be cleared of incorrect programming from childhood, society, or other patterns. Information received from an occluded subconscious will always have a bias or predisposition. Some may think that psychics, "light workers," or spiritual teachers have the truth, but, in my experience, I have seen that many bring in their psychic visions or version of truth through the lens of a clouded personal subconscious. That's why when one is seeking a psychic or reader it is important to find someone who has done therapy work, ideally shadow work, and follows some sort of spiritual path (which is not rigid or dogmatic). Those who have become purified of their own ego distortions are more proficient and accurate when tapping into truth. One can tune into the luminous or upper spheres of wisdom and connect with our higher self to receive accurate information. In addition to therapeutic and spiritual practices, it's important to raise your vibration to a higher frequency that is above all the noise "out there."

If you want to connect to the universe, think in terms of frequency, vibration, and energy, as Nikola Tesla suggested. He also recommended that we break through the denser vibrations coming at us from lower vibratory energies and channels.

Improving Intuition

In order to improve one's intuition, the key is to come from a place of neutrality. That means that the personal ego or subconscious needs to be purified, clear, or at least neutral. Neutrality or clarity with intuition means not having a preference, especially with predicting outcomes with something like politics. If one is already leaning one way or has a preference, that's going to taint the clear vision or clear sense of the truth.

But if one has done work on their subconscious and comes from a place of neutrality, they will be able to access true intuition. Developing intuition is like building a muscle, it will get stronger the more you work it out, as in practice it on friends, open-minded family members, or others, and of course try it out on yourself. When people come back to you and tell you the accuracy of your reading or psychic hit, that helps build confidence, and pushes one to practice more. In my 30+ years of doing readings, I am encouraged by clients who return over the years, and inform me about the accuracy of my previous predictions. If I wasn't delivering messages that provided healing to my clients, I would have stopped doing it years ago. Modalities that can help in developing intuition or fine tuning psychic senses are pendulums, Tarot cards, and other divination cards or tools. However, many who are pursuing a path of intuition or developing extra sensory perceptions tend to admit that the trickiest person to read for is oneself. You have to treat yourself like a client you are reading for and depersonalize the whole process. This is when the test for neutrality is challenged as one must sidestep ego and subconscious blocks or preferences, to get accurate insights.

What is intuition?

The definition of intuition from the dictionary is: "the ability to understand something immediately, without the need for conscious reasoning." Intuition can be defined with a philosophical slant as "A form of direct knowledge or insight that does not rely on logical inference or empirical evidence." Or a more spiritual interpretation is "A deep inner knowing or guidance believed to come from a higher source, such as the soul, the universe, or divine inspiration." This spiritual interpretation aligns with the meaning of intuition, and thus I refer to it as inner wisdom, higher knowing, and divine guidance.

Other ways to view intuition is through a gut feeling or instinctual impulse which hits suddenly and offers insight into a certain situation or decision. Sometimes intuition comes in very unexpected ways, such as an aversion to go somewhere at a certain time. Having a "sixth sense" is another way intuition is described, as is having a "hunch," something that guides one to take action, or feel out a situation. Sudden insights or perceptions that come out of seemingly nowhere and differ from normal thinking patterns can be forms of intuitive knowing. Intuition can come in flashes of premonition or presentiments, which are foreshadowings of things to come that then prove accurate. Intuition has also been categorized as divination, ESP, clairvoyance, clairaudience, clairsentience, and claircognition. Divination is a practice of foreseeing or predicting future events or discovering hidden knowledge through mystical or spiritual methods. It often involves interpreting signs, symbols, or omens. Tools such as Tarot cards, pendulum, scrying, the I Ching, or Runes, are used in divination practices. In a religious or spiritual context divination can be a ritualistic practice aimed at receiving guidance from deities, spirits, or cosmic forces. Psychologically, divination can be viewed as a way for individuals to tap into their subconscious mind, using symbols to gain personal insight.

ESP means "extra sensory perception," a term used in the early 20th century to describe psychic phenomenon. I remember as a youngster during the 1970s there were plenty of books out there on ESP including *Test Your ESP*, published in 1969 by the Institute for Parapsychology, *ESP: A Personal Memoir*, by Rosalind Heywood published in 1964, and, of course, the classic, *Edgar Cayce on ESP*, published in

1969 by Association for Research on Enlightenment (A.R.E.). A.R.E. is a non-profit organization founded by Edgar Cayce in 1931, dedicated to exploring topics like spirituality, holistic health, and psychic phenomena through the vast collection of psychic readings Cayce provided while in a self-induced trance state. Cayce was known as the "sleeping prophet," and brought psychic phenomena as well as past life and soul readings into the public awareness throughout the 20th century until he died in January 1945.

The Four Main Clairs

The four main clairs of intuition are **clairvoyance** (clear seeing), **clairaudience** (clear hearing), **clairsentience** (clear feeling), and **claircognizance** (clear knowing). These are all modalities or expressions of intuition – known in Sanskrit as four primary *siddhis* (spiritual gifts and mystical abilities).

Clairvoyance is the ability to perceive events beyond normal sensory contact, such as those occurring at a distance or in the future. As a form of ESP, it enables individuals to gain insight into the unseen without relying on the five physical senses. In a mystical context, clairvoyance is often linked to heightened perception, spiritual insight, or visions from other realms.

Some people have a prominent clair, while the others are latent. Clairvoyants historically are mystics such as Saint Hildegard of Bingen, a German Benedictine Abbess and Doctor of the Church, who lived 1000 years ago and had intense and prophetic visions. She wrote a work called *Scivias*, which described 26 of her visions. St. Joan of Arc claimed to have experienced visions and heard voices from angels and saints starting around the age of 13. She believed these divine messengers guided her to aid France during the Hundred Years' War.

Throughout my life I have experienced all four. When I was young I was clairvoyant and would have clear visions or dreams, and later when I started doing psychic readings I would see images and watch the movie unfold for my client. After about a decade into doing readings, clairaudience and claircognitive abilities took over as I would hear the person's story being told to me in my field and have instantaneous knowing what to say to them, which proved to be accurate. During my 30s as a hands-on healer, my clairsentience kicked in as I would feel what was happening in my client's body, and be guided to put my hands on that area and transmit healing. After almost four decades of doing readings, the clairsentience is strong when I do mediumistic work, and most of my psychic readings are clairaudient and claircognitive in nature, where clairvoyance has taken a back seat.

As I mentioned earlier, some are born with the gift of intuition, some express it at a younger age, but most of us have it as a latent ability. Sanskrit mantras can certainly enhance our intuitive faculties, whether they show up as clairvoyance, clairaudience, claircognizance, or clairsentience

In my years of chanting Sanskrit mantras and doing readings, it is my experience that all and any mantras will enhance our intuition. The caveat is that they need to be chanted consistently, correctly, and abundantly. Chanting any deity mantra will activate the *siddhis* including latent psychic or intuitive abilities.

The deities that I have found to be particularly helpful for activating extra sensory perceptions are Ganesha and Goddess Saraswati. Ganesha is powerful to remove obstacles and blocks to our intuitive powers, whether they are psychological, physiological, or karmic. Certain blockages in the chakras and *nadis* can hinder access to the higher chakras of the throat, third eye, and crown centers which tap us into Source or Divine energies. Chanting to Ganesha will ease up those blockages. Saraswati is the principle of divine speech and intelligence. The Saraswati principle activates supreme knowledge, **vidya**. Saraswati is referred to as "Maha Vidya" meaning transcendental knowledge (or great wisdom), and "Maha Vani" the transcendental word. Also called "Arya" or noble one, she also bestows blessings as "Kamadhenu," the wish-fulfilling cow, and "Dhameshwari," the diversity of wealth. She is considered to be the knowledge and the power behind the creation of the cosmos, as well as mind and sound. Goddess Saraswati bestows blessings related to communication, education, music, the arts, and gives mantras their power. Invoking Saraswati will activate the higher chakras of the Vishuda (throat), Ajna (third eye) and

Sahasrara (crown) to access clairaudience, clairvoyance, claircognizance, and Divine intuition associated with those chakras.

It is important for the modern practitioner of mantras to understand the significance of Saraswati mantras. According to Thomas Ashley-Farrand, "the Saraswati principle governs all spiritual pursuits as in the ancient scriptures. Spiritual teachers and Gurus transmit the power of mantra through the Saraswati principle. Followers of the path of Intellectual Understanding and Power of the Mind are similarly governed by this principle. The transmission of powerful *shakti* in famous gurus such as Yogananda was governed by the Saraswati principle."*

Anyone on the path to develop or enhance intuitive, psychic, or extrasensory perceptions should dive into Saraswati mantras. As I mentioned, Saraswati gives mantras their power, endows them as divine speech, and activates the *nadis* and centers of the upper chakras in the throat and brain centers.

* Thomas Ashley-Farrand, *The Ancient Power of Sanskrit Mantra and Ceremony*, vol. 2 (Saraswati Publications 2002), 218.

om eka dantaya namaha

Om Ek-ka Dan-ta-ya Nahm-ah-ha

Om – Sacred sound
Eka – One
Danta – Tusk
Ya – To the one
Namaha – I bow

Salutations to the one-tusked Lord (Ganesha), symbolizing sacrifice and strength.

This mantra invokes Ganesha, the remover of obstacles, patron of beginnings, intellect, and wisdom. This mantra gives specific reference to his one tusk, Ekadanta which symbolizes non-duality, or wholeness. It also brings resilience and adaptability, on the way to unifying body, mind, and spirit.

"Ekadanta refers to one tusk in the elephant face, which means God broke the duality and made you to have a one-pointed mind. Whoever has that oneness of mind and single-minded devotion will achieve everything."*

* Sadguru Sant Keshavadas, *Lord Ganesha* (Vishwa Dharma Publications, 1988), 32.

As with all Ganesha mantras, chanting "Om Ekadantaya Namaha" before launching a project, journey, or creative endeavor helps clear mental, emotional, and energetic obstacles. In particular, this mantra supports access to intuition and deepens connection with the higher self.

Reciting this mantra also helps dissolve inner blocks and overcome self-doubt, fear, or confusion, especially when seeking to connect with your intuitive self.

This mantra can be integrated into a broader spiritual practice or used as an invocation at the beginning with the following mantras in a sequence designed to cultivate intuition. It helps align the practitioner with divine will and fosters a deeper connection to the subtle energy body.

At times, I've included this mantra to my regular Sanskrit invocation before offering an astrology or psychic reading. I've noticed that when I chant "Om Ekadantaya Namaha" prior to a reading, I'm able to tune in more directly to the core of my client's concern. Intuitive insights come more easily, and the clarity it brings often helps to ease their anxiety around the issue.

om gaja karnakaya namaha

Om Ga-ja Kar-na-ka-ya Nahm-ah-ha

Om – Sacred sound
Gaja – Elephant
Karnakaya – One who has ears like an elephant
Namaha – I bow

Salutations to the one with elephant-like ears (Lord Ganesha).

About this mantra, Sadguru Sant Keshavadas wrote, "One can sit anywhere and tune this cosmic television (the body) with seven channels (chakras), and all 72,000 *nadis*, to any *loka* and be able to hear ancestors, angels, the voice of God, or the voice of the prophets."*

Gaja Karnakaya is another name and form of Lord Ganesha, specifically honoring his large, sensitive ears, which symbolize attentiveness, discernment, and the ability to truly listen. This mantra invokes the aspect of Ganesha that is finely attuned to subtle sound, vibration, and inner guidance. His elephant ears represent keen spiritual listening, wise discrimination, and open receptivity.

When we chant this mantra and access Ganesha's elephant ears, we are blessed with spiritual hearing,

* Sadguru Sant Keshavadas, *Lord Ganesha* (Vishwa Dharma Publications, 1988), 32.

enlightened understanding, and an open, receptive soul. By chanting this mantra we honor Ganesha calling upon his *siddhis* of deep listening, intuition, and perception on the spiritual path, and especially when we use these gifts to serve others. This is a wonderful mantra to chant before meditation or inner work. It will heighten receptivity to guidance, divine messages, and activating the gift of clairaudience.

This mantra pairs beautifully with other mantras like "Om Ekadantaya Namaha" or "Om Eim Saraswatiyei Swaha" to open the gateways to cosmic wisdom, enhance one's intuition, and receive the blessings and *darshan* of Ganesha.

I've begun integrating this mantra into my regular Sanskrit invocation before offering astrology or psychic readings. Each time I include "Om Gaja Karnakaya Namaha," I feel a deeper alignment with divine guidance, as though a clear channel opens. I'm gently led straight to the core of what my client is seeking, and the intuitive messages that come through often bring them comfort, clarity, and a sense of peace.

This is a mantra I share with those who wish to awaken and deepen their intuition, often in sacred pairing with "Om Eim Saraswatiyei Namaha." Over the years, I've received many heartfelt accounts of profound inner shifts, mystical experiences, and moments of divine insight arising from its practice. Many also share that it brings vivid, precognitive dreams that offer intuitive guidance – often later confirmed by real-life events.

Om Eim Saraswatiyei Swaha

Om I'm Sa-ras-wa-tee-yay Swa-ha

Om – Sacred sound
Eim – Seed sound of Saraswati
Saraswatiyei – To Saraswati (in dative case)
Swaha – An offering or invocation (literally: "so be it" or "I offer this")

I invoke and offer myself to Goddess Saraswati, the embodiment of wisdom and learning.

Foundation or *mula* mantra to Saraswati, goddess of Divine wisdom. Governs all spiritual pursuits, gives mantras their power. Good for education, musical and artistic endeavors and makes any project successful.

The seed mantra "Eim" was introduced in chapter 1. It honors the primordial Feminine principle that governs divine wisdom and speech, and gives Sanskrit mantras their power. Saraswati rules over artistic and scientific endeavors, music, and education. This mantra activates the Saraswati principle which gives mantras their power as magical speech.

The initial mantra I recommend for enhancing intuition, illuminating your intellect, and following divine guidance is the Saraswati seed or *bija* mantra, "Eim." The beauty of chanting "Eim" is in its simplicity and ease of pronunciation because it is a one word *bija* mantra. "Eim" is instilled with all the energies of the Saraswati precept of Divine wisdom. This mantra activates the Saraswati essence which gives mantras their power and imbues them with magical speech, as does "Om Eim Saraswatiyei Swaha."

Both mantras can be applied for successful outcomes in many situations that require the use of right speech and knowledge. It is a great aid when studying and taking tests and exams. Traditionally, in India, parents have chanted to Saraswati on behalf of their children so they would be blessed in all educational endeavors at all ages, including getting into the desired school and college or university. It is helpful to chant before a stressful event such as a job interview, a job review, a presentation, drivers test, or any other circumstance when one has to give correct answers or respond appropriately. Saraswati will put the right words on your tongue. Musicians, actors, entertainers, and presenters can chant this mantra to help with performance and stage presence.

Over the years as a consulting astrologer, I've had the privilege of working with several actors. One mantra I often recommend to them is "Om Eim Saraswatiyei Swaha," as it powerfully supports articulate speech and deepens their expressive presence on stage and screen. Many of these actors are also engaged in spiritual growth, and this mantra helps them attune more deeply to their intuition, enriching not just their craft, but all areas of their lives.

om hamsa vahinyei namaha

Om Ham-sa Va-heen-yay Nahm-ah-ha

Om – Sacred sound
Hamsa – Refers to the swan, a mystical bird in Indian philosophy that symbolizes discernment, purity, wisdom, and the breath of life (*prana*). The swan is believed to be capable of separating milk from water, a metaphor for discriminative wisdom (*viveka*).
Vahini – One who rides or is carried by
Yei – Activates shakti
Namaha – I bow

Salutations to the one (Divine Feminine) who rides the swan.

This mantra refers to Goddess Saraswati, the goddess of wisdom, speech, learning, music, and intuition, who is traditionally depicted riding a white swan. It enhances discernment and wisdom as it activates Saraswati's energies of refined intellect and insight. It is ideal for students, teachers, artists, writers, and truth seekers. Chanting it before meditation is especially supportive, as it cultivates inner stillness. The swan, *hamsa*, is linked to the breath – its name echoing the sounds of inhalation and exhalation – making this mantra a powerful complement to breathwork. It awakens the higher mind, *buddhi*, allowing one to rise above mental noise and connect with intuitive, inspired insight. This mantra harmonizes **Vach** Shakti, the subtle power behind speech. Saraswati is also known as *Vach*, the giver of eloquence and expression. Chanting this mantra purifies communication, making it more refined, impactful, and graceful. It serves as an invocation of Saraswati's grace, inviting her presence into creative, intellectual, and spiritual pursuits.

I recommended the mantra "Om Hamsa Vahinyei Namaha" to my client Josh, who faced a major career crossroads. He had one week to decide whether to take a new job – far better pay and benefits, but requiring frequent public speaking, which terrified him.

Torn and uncertain, Josh spiraled in indecision, stuck in endless mental loops. I told him to stop analyzing and chant "Om Hamsa Vahinyei Namaha" 108 times a day for a week – without thinking about the choice. This mantra activates divine intelligence and clear communication.

He followed through and soon dropped into deep meditation, feeling calm and assured. One day, the phrase "Learn German" arose in his mind – random, he thought.

By the third day, his confidence returned. By Monday, he knew the new job wasn't just better – it felt right. When he accepted, his employer said, "Great – hope you can speak German! We're opening a Frankfurt office."

Josh was floored. The mantra hadn't just cleared his mind – it had prepared him for what was ahead.

sat chid ekam brahma

Sat Chit Ek-am Bra-ma

Om – Sacred sound
Sat – Truth, Existence, Eternal Being
Chid – Consciousness, Awareness
Ekam – One, Non-Dual, Unity
Brahma – The Absolute Supreme Reality

The one absolute reality is truth and consciousness.

This mantra serves as a powerful catalyst to initiate or accelerate the process of accumulating true knowledge. It supports the attainment of deeper meditative states, intuitive clarity, inner knowing, and a felt connection to the greater whole.

By attuning to the pure field of *Sat* (being) and *Chid* (awareness) – the fundamental essence of the universe and the Higher Self – it dissolves ego-identification and aligns you with clarity, presence, and truth.

This is a potent and intense mantra – one that may not resonate with everyone. In my experience, it has guided me into deep meditative states, helping me access the core of my inquiries and strengthen my connection to Source. Simply chanting it often draws me effortlessly into trance-like stillness. It's especially powerful when chanted before sleep, as it can open the gateway to deeper, more meaningful dream states. I have experienced very vivid dreams that I was able to remember when chanting "Sat Chid Ekam Brahma" before falling asleep.

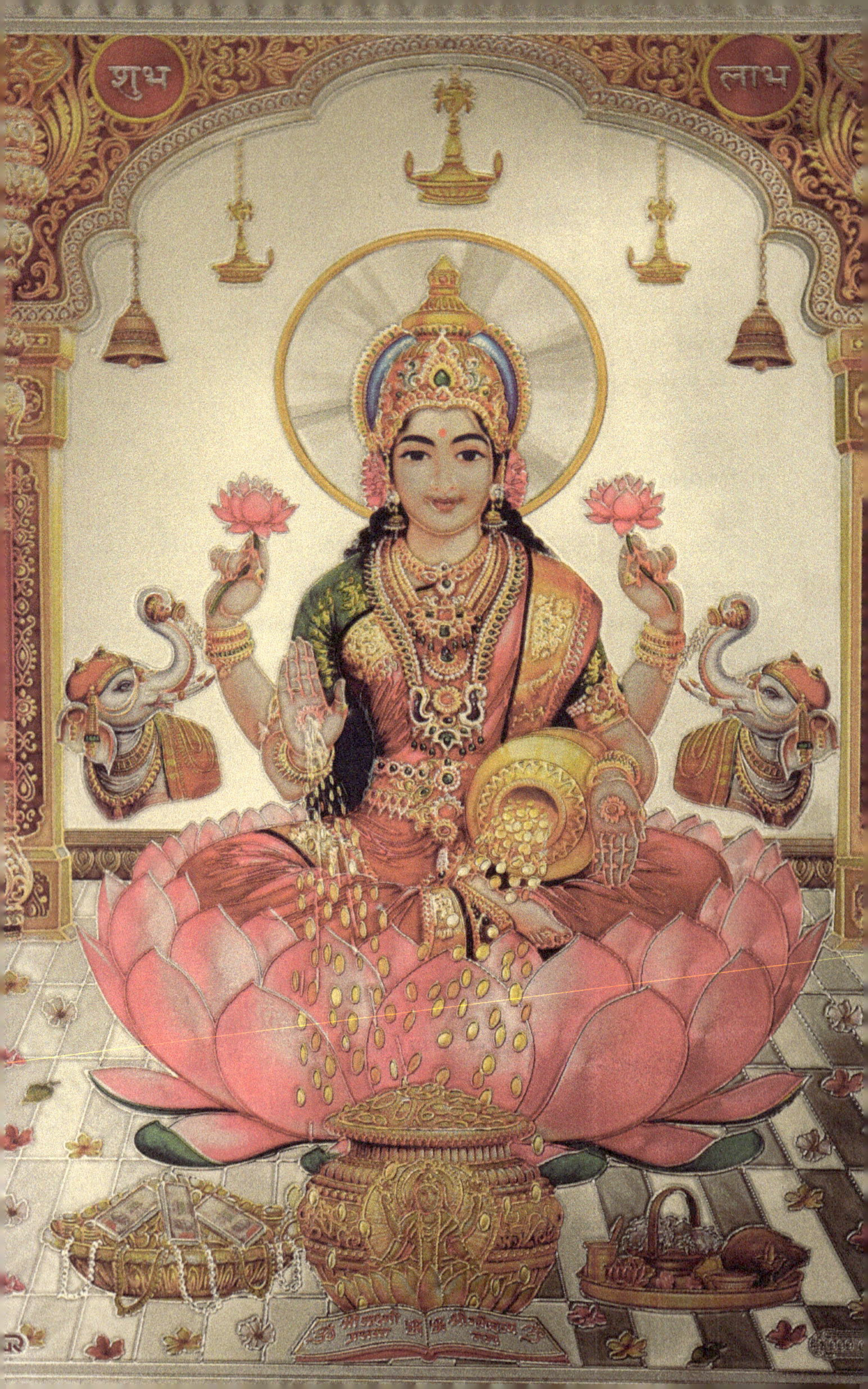
शुभ
लाभ

5

Mantras for Prosperity

The Lakshmi Principle

In the Vedic pantheon, Lakshmi is the goddess of abundance, prosperity, and auspiciousness, revered as the embodiment of divine grace and beauty. She is the *shakti* (dynamic power) of Narayana – the sustaining force of the universe – and the divine consort of Vishnu, the Preserver. Together, Lakshmi and Vishnu represent the balance of cosmic preservation and nourishment, and are often invoked for blessings of both spiritual and material wealth.

Lakshmi's energy sustains life itself. She is called upon to dispel scarcity, stagnation, and misfortune, and to replace them with flow, vitality, and blessings. Her presence brings not only financial stability, but also health as wealth, harmonious relationships, elevated status, fertility, and the joy of good children. True prosperity, in Lakshmi's realm, extends far beyond money – it encompasses all forms of well-being and fulfillment.

As the divine feminine, Lakshmi symbolizes the *shakti* that enlivens, nurtures, and beautifies existence. Inviting her into the home is a sacred act of aligning with the feminine principle that sustains life with creativity, elegance, and serenity. She governs the qualities of beauty, grace, and inner harmony, and her presence sanctifies the household with peace, abundance, and spiritual richness.

In traditional Indian homes, Goddess Lakshmi is lovingly invoked to invite prosperity, fortune, and spiritual well-being. As the deity of both material and spiritual wealth, her presence is believed to attract financial stability, opportunity, and a steady flow of resources into the household.

Beyond wealth, Lakshmi nurtures domestic harmony. Her energy fosters a peaceful, balanced environment that supports loving relationships and emotional well-being. Invoking her is not only a prayer for abundance, but also a call to uphold *dharma* – right conduct, cleanliness, and reverence for sacred space – all of which welcome and sustain her blessings.

Homes are kept clean and filled with light, as Lakshmi is said to dwell where beauty and order prevail. Offerings of flowers, sweets, and daily chants of her mantras – especially on Fridays, the day dedicated to her – are ways devotees honor her presence.

Bringing Lakshmi into the home is a devotional act of alignment with the energies of grace, abundance, and sacred prosperity, allowing her blessings to flow not only through the material plane, but into the very heart of one's daily life.

Prosperity

Prosperity is a highly sought-after topic, as many people eagerly look for guidance on which mantras to chant for financial growth. In my readings and sessions, the top three areas clients seek clarity on are relationships, money, and health. Naturally, depending on the current economic climate, money takes priority. The great news is that Sanskrit mantras can be powerful tools to cultivate a wealth-conscious mindset and help clear limiting beliefs and energetic blocks that hinder manifestation.

In my experience, Sanskrit mantras help with clearing out blocks or obstacles that subconsciously limit the attraction of money. Ganesha mantras are very effective in clearing blocks about money, especially the mantra "Om Lakshmi Ganapatayei Namaha" (covered in chapter 3), which removes blockages or limiting beliefs to personal prosperity. It is supportive to address the subconscious with other modalities to find out what the money mindset is that usually has been gestating since youth due to one's circumstances financially during childhood and formative years. Lack of self worth is a common issue that can interfere with prosperity in life, and is usually rooted in childhood experiences. It can be helpful to work with a therapist or certified money mindset or wealth coach to weed out limiting subconscious beliefs around money. I worked with wealth coach, Therese Nicklas, (wealthcoachforwomen.com) and found it a nice adjunct to chanting Sanskrit mantras for prosperity.

It's beneficial to align your consciousness with abundance and wealth instead of scarcity or lack. In today's world, this mindset shift can be crucial to rising above the chaos and collective fears around the economy. No matter what's happening externally, nurturing an inner sense of abundance and prosperity is vital. Many people have created significant wealth even during difficult economic times, so it's important to let go of the belief that your prosperity depends on external circumstances. According to the prosperity laws of various metaphysical teachings, when you change your mind, you change your results.

As Joseph Murphy wrote: "God is the giver and the gift, man is the receiver. God dwells in man, and this means that the treasure house of infinite riches is within you and all around you. By learning the laws of the mind, you can extract from the infinite storehouse within you everything you need in order to live gloriously, joyously, and abundantly."* Traditionally, affirmations have been recommended to undo negative programs or change mental programming around prosperity.

Some examples of affirmations that may work for you include: *"I trust the Universal spirit of Prosperity to provides richly for me now." "My source is a source of plenty, and I receive all I desire and require and more." "I am open to receive all the blessings the Universe has for me now, and the Universe sends unlimited resources."*

* Joseph Murphy Joseph Murphy, *Your Infinite Power to be Rich* (Parker Publishing Co., 1966), 28.

I've read many self-help books on prosperity consciousness and found them very valuable, including the pioneering works in prosperity ideology of Catherine Ponder and Florence Scovel Shinn which shared prosperity affirmations and demonstrations of manifestation. In fact, I read these decades before I discovered the power of Sanskrit mantras for prosperity. Catherine Ponder, a Unity Minister, wrote some pivotal books in the positive thought and new consciousness movement during the 1960s and 1970s including *The Secret of Unlimited Prosperity*, *The Dynamic Laws of Prosperity*, *Open Your Mind to Prosperity*, and *The Prospering Power of Love*. It may be helpful to read these books to understand more about affirmations.

Affirmations are certainly a good adjunct to chanting Sanskrit, but they may not be able to fully bypass the subconscious blocks, because they aren't spoken in a vibrational language as is Sanskrit. As described earlier, the advantage of chanting in Sanskrit is that it can raise our vibration both mentally and palpably. The Sanskrit language is a tool for working with the subtle energy potential, represented by each of the hundreds of chakras within the energetic body. Sanskrit mantras for prosperity are a wonderful technique to shift your vibration, and change subconscious patterns that may interfere with attracting more prosperity. Some of my students tell me that by chanting the mantras I have given them, they have cleared issues around self worth and deservedness.

Om Shrim Maha Lakshmiyei Namaha

Om Shreem Mah-ha Laksh-mee-yei Nahm-ah-ha

Om – Sacred sound
Shrim – Seed sound of Lakshmi (abundance, beauty, prosperity)
Maha – Great
Lakshmiyei – To Lakshmi (feminine, dative form)
Namaha – I bow

I offer my respectful salutations to the great Goddess Lakshmi, the source of all abundance and prosperity.

This mantra is the *mula*, or foundational, mantra dedicated to Lakshmi, the Goddess of Prosperity. It honors the Divine Feminine principle of abundance, with the sacred seed sound "Shrim," embodying this powerful energy. Chanting this mantra invokes the blessings of Goddess Lakshmi to bring material wealth, financial stability, and a general sense of abundance into one's life.

By reciting it, one invites Lakshmi to enter the home, ensuring continued prosperity, grace, and ease in the pursuit of worldly goals. The mantra calls upon her to assist with all forms of prosperity – not only material riches but also spiritual wealth, sufficient nourishment, blessings for family and children, meaningful employment, beauty, pleasure, and the precious gift of time to cultivate a spiritual life. In this way, it fosters spiritual abundance alongside worldly success.

Invoking Lakshmi through this sacred vibration also awakens compassion, empathy, maternal love, and the effortless flow of spiritual wisdom. Regular chanting may bring improved education, fulfilling work that one eagerly embraces, and increased financial reward.

On a deeper level, the mantra supports spiritual growth, emotional balance, and peace of mind. Its repetition purifies the subtle energy field, attracts positive vibrations, and helps dissolve obstacles rooted in scarcity consciousness or financial stress. The vibrational power of the mantra sharpens concentration, calms the mind, and aligns the practitioner with the divine frequency of grace and abundance.

Lakshmi reveals herself to the noble-hearted seeker of truth – those who chant her mantra with steadfast devotion and regularity – bringing blessings that nurture both material success and spiritual fulfillment.

One of the very first mantras Namadeva recommended I chant was "Om Shrim Maha Lakshmiyei Namaha." Around the same time, I discovered through my Vedic astrology chart that Lakshmi was the ideal deity to invoke, as my chart is ruled by Venus – the planet associated with Lakshmi's divine energy. Embracing this mantra wholeheartedly, I soon witnessed remarkable shifts in my life.

Opportunities began to appear seemingly out of nowhere. People gifted me jewelry, flowers, concert tickets, and other tokens of pleasure – items all closely aligned with

Lakshmi's domain of beauty, abundance, and grace. My friend Shivani, inspired by this energy, began crafting malas, and I was a grateful recipient of her exquisite creations.

Speaking of my friend Shivani Silvia Sune, founder of Shakti Malas – her former company specializing in hand-crafted malas – she shares an inspiring story about chanting this mantra: "Jill invited me to a special prosperity workshop at Kripalu led by Namadeva, focused on the blessings of Lakshmi. I longed to attend with my daughter Lalita but didn't have the $2,000 needed. So I began chanting the Maha Lakshmi mantra – 'Om Shrim Maha Lakshmiyei Namaha' – with heartfelt prayer: 'Lakshmi, please bring me $2,000 so I can attend.' A few days later, a client at the Fontainebleau Hotel ordered dozens of malas. The payment totaled exactly $2,000 – the precise amount I had asked for. This manifestation amazed me and reaffirmed the grace of Lakshmi and the power of sincere mantra practice. I was deeply grateful to Jill for guiding me to this path and to Namadeva for the workshop where I received my initiation into the Lakshmi mantra – a truly transformative experience."

om suvarna dayei namaha

Om Su-var-na Da-yei Nahm-ah-ha

Om – Sacred sound
Suvarna – Gold or "golden" - symbolizing purity, preciousness, and radiant abundance
Dayei – Giver (feminine form)
Namaha – I bow

I offer my respectful salutations to the great Goddess Lakshmi, the source of all abundance and prosperity.

This is a Lakshmi mantra invoking her as the Divine Mother who generously bestows wealth and golden blessings upon her votaries. It specifically asks for tangible material wealth in the form of money. This mantra is a heartfelt invocation to Lakshmi as the Divine Mother, the benevolent bestower of wealth and golden blessings. Lakshmi has been revered for millennia across the Indian subcontinent as the embodiment of abundance, prosperity, and good fortune. Often depicted seated on a lotus flower, she symbolizes purity, spiritual power, and the unfolding of inner and outer wealth. As the consort of Vishnu, the preserver deity, Lakshmi's blessings are seen as essential for sustaining both worldly success and spiritual harmony. Historically, Lakshmi has been honored not only as the goddess of wealth but as a protector of family, a guardian of fertility, and a guide to spiritual enlightenment. The symbolism of gold within this mantra reflects the sacred qualities of durability, purity, and radiant light – qualities that Lakshmi bestows upon her devotees to illuminate their path to fulfillment and joy.

Chanting this mantra cultivates prosperity and strengthens financial stability while nurturing an open-hearted spirit of giving and receiving. It aligns the practitioner with the abundant flow of the Divine Mother's benevolent energy, fostering both material success and spiritual grace. This mantra is chanted to attract financial abundance from both expected and unforeseen sources. "Om Suvarna Dayei Namaha" clear blockages rooted in scarcity consciousness and invites a steady flow of blessings. It opens doors to new opportunities and nurtures positive relationships. Its effectiveness is heightened when one cultivates a focused intention on wealth, success, and compassionate generosity before chanting.

As a facilitator for many years guiding groups in Sanskrit mantra chanting, this particular mantra has been one of the most frequently requested for prosperity. Participants often describe feeling pleasant sensations flowing through their bodies and seeing golden light surrounding themselves and the entire room.

Namadeva explained that this golden hue represents the highest vibrational frequency for healing, and those who carry it are natural healers. Beyond its uplifting energy, many group members have also reported unexpected financial blessings and good fortune after chanting it.

om shrim klim namah shivaya

Om Shreem Kleem Nahm-ah-ha Shi-vah-yah

Om – Sacred sound
Shrim – Abundance, beauty (Lakshmi's seed sound)
Klim – Attraction, magnetic power (associated with Divine Love)
Namah Shivaya – I bow to Shiva (sacred five-syllable mantra)

I bow to Lord Shiva, invoking both abundance and divine attraction.

by Dr. Alexi Jardine Martel

"Om Shrim Klim Namah Shivaya" is known as an abundance mantra; it provides the chanter with both material and spiritual abundance. The mantra combines the foundational Shiva mantra "Om Namah Shivaya" with the seed sounds "Shrim" and "Klim." "Om Namah Shivaya," discussed in detail later in the chapter on Liberation mantras, is a powerful mantra for evolving consciousness. The foundation Shiva mantra is considered to have a masculine energy, as the archetype of pure consciousness represented by Shiva is typically considered masculine in the Vedic tradition. Conversely most seed sounds including "Shrim" and "Klim" are considered feminine as they are concentrated energetic expressions of *shakti*. Together the masculine force of Shiva

(Consciousness) and the feminine force of Shakti (Energy) interact to produce the entire universe. "Om Shrim Klim Namah Shivaya" combines both archetypal forces into one very powerful mantra. The interaction of the masculine and feminine energies in one mantra increases the power of each part of the mantra, as here the sum of the parts is more than the individual components. Just as the interaction of male and female creates new physical life, the interaction of the archetypal masculine and spiritual forces breathes new life into the chanter and transforms them and their circumstances to something greater than before.

This mantra tends to attract abundance in a manner similar to other abundance mantras such as the foundational Lakshmi mantra. The seed sound "Shrim" is considered the seed sound of Lakshmi, the feminine principle of abundance. Combined with the seed sound of attraction "Klim," which amplifies the effect, the mantra blesses the chanter with great abundance. Abundance in the Vedic spiritual tradition can mean many things. Certainly the chanter can invoke the energies of the mantra with a specific form of abundance in mind (health, financial wealth, new friendships, new romantic relationships, a new job, a new car, etc.). The mantra will respond to the heartfelt desire of the chanter. However, the mantra will also bless the chanter with abundance that they might not know they are lacking such as new relationships or professional opportunities, enhanced optimism, increased patience, or greater peace of mind. Like a good improv comedy act is built on the principle of "Yes, and...", abundance mantras say yes to what the chanter desires and expands from there.

I can personally vouch for the power of "Om Shrim Klim Namah Shivaya." I have completed multiple 40-day disciplines with the mantra; I felt called to chant the mantra because it resonated with me. Although I didn't embark on the spiritual disciplines with a specific goal in mind, I was open to whatever positive energies the mantra would bring into my life. During the course of my first 40-day discipline with the mantra, I secured a job as a web developer. At the time, this was somewhat unlikely because although I was finishing my undergraduate college education, I had not formally studied anything related to the technology field. I had taught myself some programming in my free time, but my formal degrees were in psychology and political science. However, I was applying for web development jobs, which admittedly was a longshot. Until I chanted the Shiva-Shakti mantra, the job application process seemed fruitless, yet during the discipline the wheels of karma began to move and I successfully applied and interviewed for a job that fit all my desires and needs at the time. Ironically, I didn't attribute the good luck around getting the job to the mantra until I reflected after the fact, as I mostly attributed it to my hard work and perseverance. Of course, two things can be true. The hard work (spending my free time in college learning web development) and the perseverance (applying for many jobs over a long period of time) were likely necessary; however, the mantra helped "grease the wheels" of karma in just the right way so that my efforts were richly rewarded. Mantras often add the luck factor that, when combined with focused personal effort toward one's object of desire, grants great success. The combination of spiritual practices with practical effort is key. Just as a purely materialistic approach to life with no consideration of the mystical might lead to an impoverished spirit and limited success, so too does simply chanting and waiting around for your miracle severely limit your potential for success. We are on the physical planet for a reason and the dichotomy of material and spiritual is fundamentally based on illusion. However, while we still view these material and spiritual spheres of life as different, we should make sustained efforts on both fronts to thrive. As they say in Islam, "Trust in God, but tie up your camel."

ha sa ka la e i la hreem
ha sa ka la e i la hreem

Ha Sa Ka La Eh Ee La Hreem

Ha Sa Ka La Eh Ee La Hreem

Ha Sa Ka La – Represents elements of subtle creation
E I La – Energies of Shakti (divine feminine)
Hreem – Seed sound of divine power and transformation (associated with Mahadevi)

A sacred vibrational mantra invoking the energy of wealth, abundance, and divine transformation.

These *bija* syllables are said to stimulate prosperity vibrations and open the channels through which wealth and success flow. "Hrim," known as a powerful Shakti *bija*, represents the energy of divine illumination, transformation, and protection. It amplifies the potency of the mantra and connects the chanter to the higher spiritual energy of **Kubera**. The mantra "Ha Sa Ka La E I La Hreem" is composed of specific *bija* sounds or syllables, each carrying potent vibrational energy connected to the deity Kubera, the celestial treasurer. These sounds are believed to activate the energy centers linked to wealth and abundance within the body and consciousness.

Lord Kubera is the Hindu god of wealth, prosperity, and the treasurer of the gods. Traditionally depicted as a plump, joyful figure adorned with jewels, he holds a money pot or mongoose, symbolizing abundance. As guardian of the North, Kubera safeguards earthly riches. Invoking him attracts prosperity, financial stability, and wealth protection. Kubera works with Lakshmi to usher in prosperity and stability. The mantra attracts money swiftly, dissolves energetic blockages, and clears negativity that hinders abundance. It attunes the mind to achievement, aligning intentions with divine abundance and nurturing both outer prosperity and inner richness.

As a holistic practitioner and astrologer who depends on clients for my livelihood, Namadeva assured me that chanting to Lakshmi, along with this Kubera mantra, would bring a steady flow of clients – and he was right! For over 20 years, whenever I need to attract more clients or income, I've turned to this mantra. Unexpected sources of money, like lottery wins and surprise gifts, also appeared. Chanting it opened spiritual doors as well, including the honor of hosting Namadeva's workshops – blessings that carried deep karmic meaning. I now recommend this mantra to anyone seeking greater abundance, especially those whose work depends on attracting clients, customers, or patrons. Lakshmi and Kubera consistently bless the flow of those seeking your services.

om sham kuberaya namaha

Om Sham Ku-bay-ra-ya Nahm-ah-ha

Om – Sacred sound
Sham – Peace, auspiciousness
Kuberaya – To Kubera, the god of wealth and treasures
Namaha – I bow

Salutations to Lord Kubera, the guardian of divine wealth and prosperity.

This mantra is a sacred salutation that opens the channels to divine prosperity. It is not merely a call for material gain, but a holistic invocation seeking financial stability grounded in spiritual integrity and mindful abundance. The mantra aligns the practitioner's intentions with universal laws of wealth, encouraging generosity, balance, and gratitude alongside material success.

This mantra is a powerful invocation of Lord Kubera's blessings, inviting material wealth, financial stability, and a continuous flow of prosperity into one's life. It works to dissolve financial obstacles and clear negative energies that hinder abundance.

Through regular chanting, the practitioner's energy becomes attuned to the vibration of prosperity, amplifying the ability to manifest desires and attract new opportunities. Commonly used in rituals, meditations, and prayers centered on wealth, business success, and financial well-being, this mantra serves not only to draw external riches but also to cultivate a mindset of gratitude and mindful stewardship. In embracing this mantra, one aligns with the divine principles of abundance, fostering responsible management of resources alongside lasting prosperity.

This mantra, especially when paired with a Lakshmi mantra such as “Om Suvarna Dayei Namaha,” or even the simple seed syllable “Shrim,” is extraordinarily powerful and known for its rapid efficacy in attracting money. I have given this mantra to several clients facing financial hardship, and almost without fail, within 24 hours money appears – often in ways both expected and surprising. I affectionately call it the “fast cash mantra.”

When I first began chanting it myself, I experienced a sudden influx of payments from multiple clients – many booking not just one session, but several in advance, and even purchasing gift certificates for friends. I also incorporate visualization into my practice, imagining $100 bills before chanting. Remarkably, this often manifests in reality, with clients paying me in crisp hundred-dollar bills.

Truly, when it comes to manifesting abundance, cash is king – and this mantra is a direct gateway to inviting that flow.

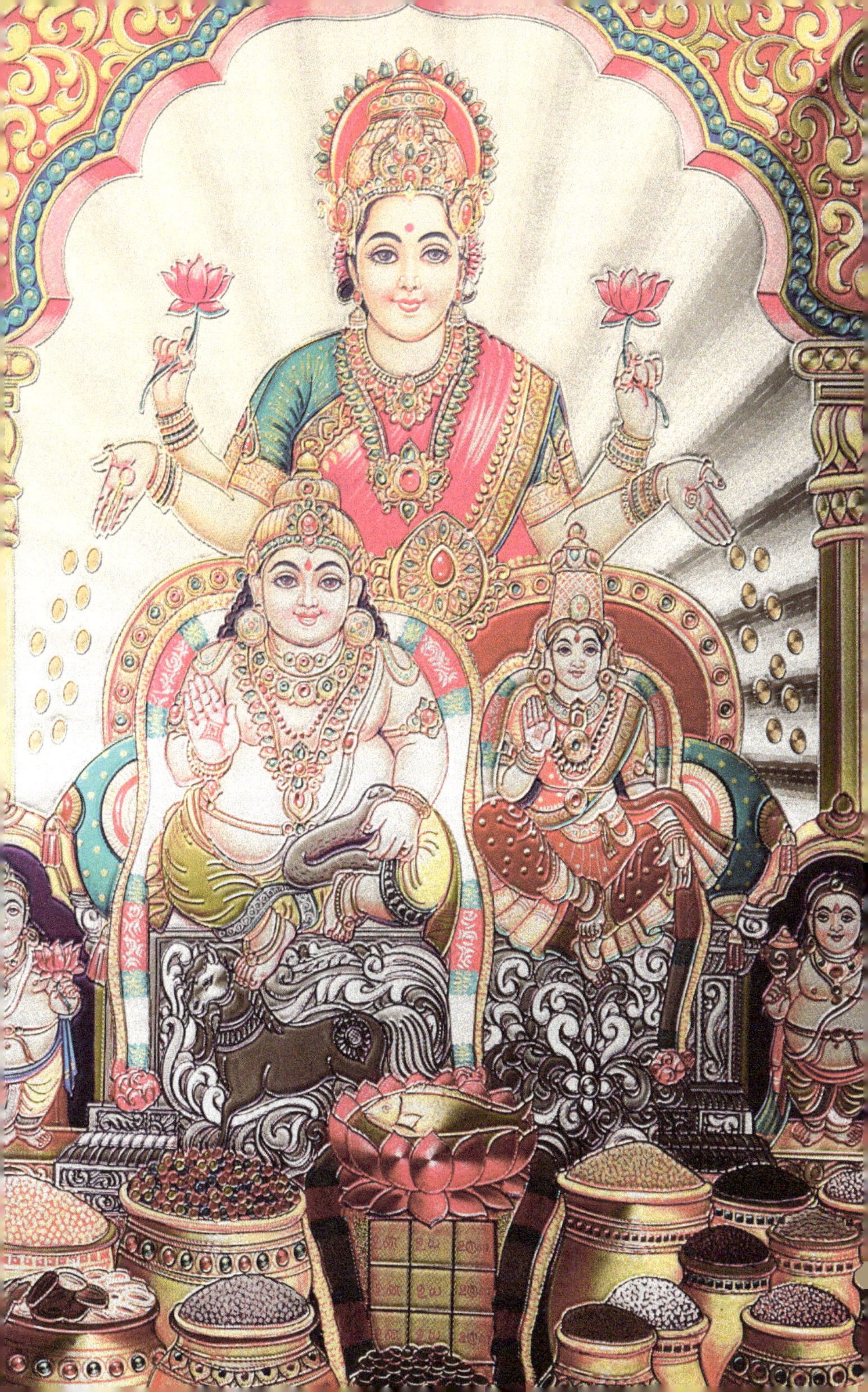

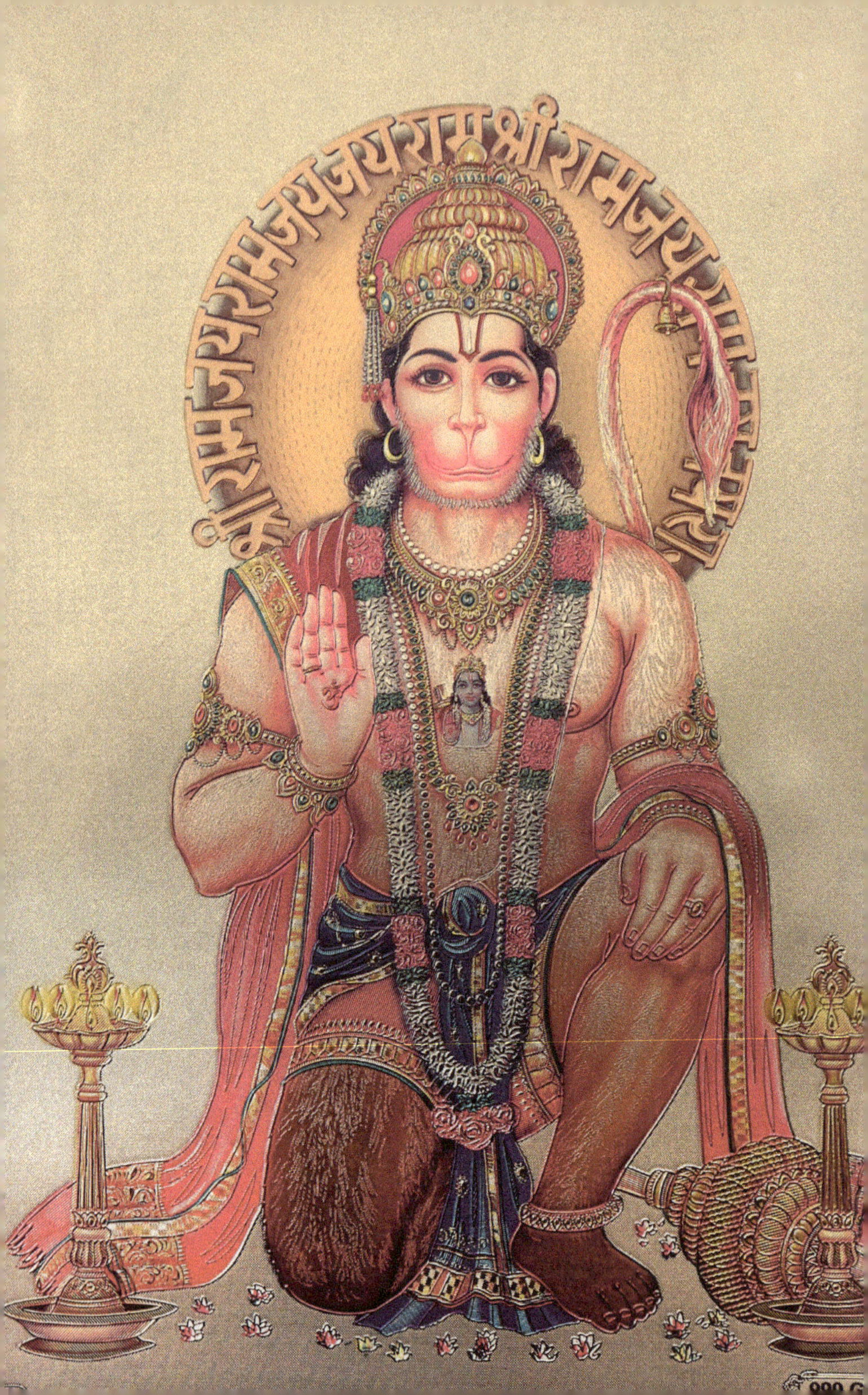
श्री राम जय राम जय जय राम श्री राम जय राम जय

6
Mantras for Healing

The Ram and Hanuman Principles

Ram, in the Vedic pantheon of deities, is revered as an incarnation of Vishnu, the preserver within the male **Trimurti**. He is best known as the noble hero of the epic Ramayana, where he embodies *dharma* – the cosmic law that upholds virtue, righteousness, and order in the universe. Ram represents the ideal of divine kingship and stands as a timeless symbol of moral integrity, truthfulness, loyalty, and unwavering devotion to duty.

Ram is invoked for healing because he is a solar deity, deeply connected to the Sun through his lineage in the Solar Dynasty (*Suryavansha*). As an incarnation of Vishnu, born into the *Surya Vamsa*, Ram carries the radiant qualities of the Sun (***Surya***), and his mantras channel the healing light of this celestial force.

In Vedic astrology, the Sun is seen as the giver of *prana* (life force) and is the source of divine illumination. It governs the heart, boosts immunity, supports longevity, and fosters cellular regeneration. As a solar archetype, Ram embodies these same qualities – he is the sustainer of life, the awakener of consciousness, and a potent force of healing and transformation.

To chant to Ram in Sanskrit is to align with this sacred solar fire – a divine force that illuminates, purifies, and revitalizes body, mind, and spirit.

On a physical level, Ram's energy activates **Agni**, the digestive fire in Ayurveda. A strong Agni is essential for metabolism, clarity of thought, and resistance to disease. On a mental and emotional level, Ram mantras help dissolve mental fog, depression, and self-doubt, restoring discernment, confidence, and inner clarity.

Chanting to Ram also acts as a natural purifier, much like sunlight. It helps remove both physical and energetic stagnation. In traditional healing contexts, Ram's solar vibrations are believed to support recovery from skin conditions, eye disorders, fatigue, anemia, and low immunity.

hanuman

Hanuman, the beloved monkey deity, in the Vedic tradition, is revered as the devoted servant of Lord Ram and one of the central figures in the Indian epic, the *Ramayana*. In the story, Hanuman plays a vital role in aiding Ram on his quest to rescue his wife Sita from the demon king Ravana. His heroic acts including leaping across oceans, lifting mountains, and defying death are legendary. Yet beyond these mythic feats, Hanuman stands as a profound spiritual archetype.

He is the embodiment of selfless devotion (**bhakti**), unshakable strength, fearlessness, and mastery over the mind and senses. Though often portrayed in playful or humble form, Hanuman carries immense spiritual power and serves as a bridge between the Divine and the human heart.

Spiritually, Hanuman is considered an incarnation of Lord Shiva, yet his entire being is dedicated to serving Ram, the avatar of Vishnu. In this way, Hanuman uniquely unites two great divine forces: *shakti*, the energy of dynamic power and transformation, and *bhakti*, the energy of love, devotion, and surrender. Within him, power and humility, strength and love, coexist in perfect harmony – offering a living template for the awakened, devoted soul.

The relationship between Hanuman and Ram lies at the very heart of Bhakti Yoga, the path of devotion. In this sacred dynamic, Hanuman represents *prana* – the subtle life force, the breath, and the energy of selfless service – while Ram symbolizes the *Self*, the Divine, the soul's innermost truth. Their union reflects the eternal dance between breath and spirit, action and surrender, the servant and the Beloved.

Hanuman is not only the archetype of devotion; he is the very embodiment of *prana*, the animating energy that sustains all of life. In the yogic and Ayurvedic traditions, *prana* is the key to vitality, immunity, mental clarity, and emotional resilience. When this life force is flowing freely, we feel energized, centered, and aligned with our highest purpose.

Chanting Hanuman mantras infuses the body and mind with pranic energy, helping to restore balance in the nervous system, calm the mind, and revitalize the physical body. These sacred sounds can dissolve fear, self-doubt, and internal conflict – especially in times of anxiety, emotional turbulence, or spiritual fatigue. Hanuman's vibration grounds us, stabilizes the mental field, and clears the subtle pathways where stress and fragmentation tend to accumulate. By attuning to Hanuman's presence through mantra, we are bathed in a healing current which balances emotions, strengthens the body, increases vitality, and sparks the soul's innate light.

Chanting Sanskrit mantras with the intention of healing – whether for oneself or others – is a powerful and transformative practice. These sacred sound formulas help dissolve energetic blockages in the body's subtle pathways, allowing energy to move freely and restoring natural flow. As these channels open, vitality increases and life force energy is enhanced. In yogic philosophy, *prana* is considered essential to health and vitality. Hanuman embodies this principle, representing the power of breath to energize and sustain the body. Mantra chanting can transmit healing across all layers of being: emotional, mental, physical, and spiritual.

When I chant healing mantras, I often find myself intuitively guided toward the resources I need – whether that's connecting with the right healers, discovering helpful technologies, supplements, or remedies. In particular, mantras like "Om Shrim Dhanvantre Namaha" seem to enhance this process, aligning me with tools that support my healing journey. These mantras also appear to amplify the golden, life-giving light of the sun, energizing both body and spirit.

Chanting activates my own innate healing abilities and can also invite spiritual healing guides to assist in the process, which is explained in a book entitled *M.A.P.* by Machaelle Small Wright. Chanting calms the nervous system, particularly engaging the parasympathetic response, which allows the body to rest, repair, and restore balance. Mantras also bring mental clarity, helping me discern the right steps to take – whether it involves changes in diet, the use of supplements, or exploring specific healing modalities. They encourage self-care by promoting healthier choices, establishing clear boundaries, and fostering discernment about what I take into my body and mind.

On an emotional level, chanting helps restore balance and supports deep healing. Often, physical issues are rooted in unresolved emotional wounds. Mantras offer the wisdom needed to recognize and release what irritates or unsettles us. They help identify emotional triggers, guiding us to the root cause of dis-ease. This insight can be especially powerful in overcoming depression, managing anxiety, and disrupting patterns of compulsive thinking. Mantras also help reduce fear by fostering a sense of safety and grounding.

Resilience and confidence often arise as natural byproducts of this emotional stability. Finally, chanting fosters a profound sense of spiritual connectedness – a reminder that there is a higher order at work. This awareness alone can ease anxiety, reinforcing a sense of trust in the divine flow of life.

Through my own experience, I came to understand that the solar plexus is the body's healing generator – and it was this realization that introduced me to the power of sun mantras. I vividly remember chanting sun mantras at a retreat with Namadeva in the Sierra Madre Mountains, and suddenly feeling an intense heat radiating from my solar plexus. I exclaimed, "My plexus is on fire!" Everyone around me laughed and said, "That's your sun center!" In that moment, I knew something profound was happening. I was activating and clearing deep energetic layers. It was a clear sign that my innate healing abilities were awakening. I was burning through *tapas* – the transformative inner heat – releasing old imprints and stepping more fully into my path as a healer.

These mantras are shared for educational and spiritual purposes, not as medical advice. They support personal growth and healing but should not replace professional care or guidance from a qualified healthcare provider.

om bhalachandraya namaha

Om Bha-la-Chan-dra-yah Nahm-ah-ha

Om – Sacred sound

Bhala – Forehead

Chandra – Moon

Ya – To the one who

Namaha – I bow

Salutations to the one who wears the moon on his forehead – a name for Lord Shiva.

This is one of the 18 esoteric mantras of Ganesha as taught by mantra guru Sadguru Sant Keshavadas. It is a healing mantra which activates the power of Ganapati to remove obstacles. The special blessing of this mantra is that it brings unity with Shiva, bestowing healing power. **Chandra** is the Sanskrit word for moon, specifically referring to the crescent moon in this mantra. Bhalachandra translates to that chakra from where the nectar drips. That is the secret of all healing. The nectar refers to *soma*, a sweet spiritual substance produced in the body when connecting to Divine Source, which drips from the third eye into the throat. Also referred to as *Amrita* (nectar of the Gods), it can be activated by spiritual practices and in the presence of true gurus. Chanting this mantra will produce *amrita* which is the secret of all healing. It activates powerful healing potential at the new and full moon. Sadguru Sant Keshavadas attributes this mantra as "identifying with the Truth and feeling constantly that you are carrying the crescent moon, the symbol of growth, and nectar of peace."*

This mantra can trigger deep meditations and revelations due to its activation of the third eye center. It can help clear the mind. As a Ganesha mantra it helps with the removal obstacles to healing. When chanting "Om Bhala Chandraya Namaha," the remedies, healers, or interventions needed to help with a health issue can be revealed. It provides clarity about what is needed to heal a situation or affliction. Chanting it will help to get to the root of a health issue which may reside in the emotional, mental, or physical body. It provides insights into the nature of healing in general.

I recommend this to clients who are chanting for healing. It can be used alone or preceding other mantras for those who seek health solutions. When I lead groups in chanting healing mantras, I will begin with this mantra. My students tend to get very deep into the chant process and feel like they went into altered states of consciousness when chanting this mantra. By the end of the session, they have received an inner message regarding the next step for healing, or insights into another issue.

This mantra helps one become more intuitive, but also brings in strong healing energies.

* Sadguru Sant Keshavadas, *Lord Ganesha* (Vishwa Dharma Publications, 1988), 33.

om ram ramaya namaha

Om Rahm Rahm-eye-yah Nahm-ah-ha

Om – Sacred sound
Ram – Fire, transformation (also invokes Lord Rama)
Ramaya – To Rama
Namaha – I bow

Salutations to Lord Rama, embodiment of dharma, virtue, and inner strength.

Ram is the seed sound that activates the Manipura chakra, where the body's healing generator is located. It invokes the energy of inner strength, fire, digestion (physical and spiritual), and willpower. Ram or "Hram" (a seed mantra for the sun) power-up the Manipura chakra which then emits healing to those parts of the body which need it. It's not a coincidence that the translation of the mantra is "Ram please bring healing to the Earth where it is needed." The Earth element being related to the body. Chanting "Ram" creates warmth and healing in the body which is palpable. The longer Ram mantra is "Om Ram Ramaya Namaha," which is chanted to bring in healing for body or mind.

I've recommended this mantra to clients and students for calming the mind and supporting emotional or mental healing, especially anxiety in young people. It helps quell negative self-talk, obsessive thoughts, and discursive thinking. Chanting while placing hands on areas needing healing can ignite the palm chakras, producing heat or tingling as energy transmits. It's an excellent mantra for healers before hands-on sessions.

It is easy to pronounce and works on the mind immediately. Many hands-on healers report feeling amplified healing energy flowing through their arms and hands. "Ram" or "Rama" activates the solar plexus (Manipura chakra), generating sensations of heat radiating to areas needing healing. Parents can chant it for anxious children, or children can chant themselves.

I recommended it to a young man with severe anxiety going to college in Washington, DC. He chanted "Om Ram Ramaya Namaha" before leaving and throughout his first semester. His mother later shared it helped him navigate anxiety and live like a normal college student, providing profound mental healing.

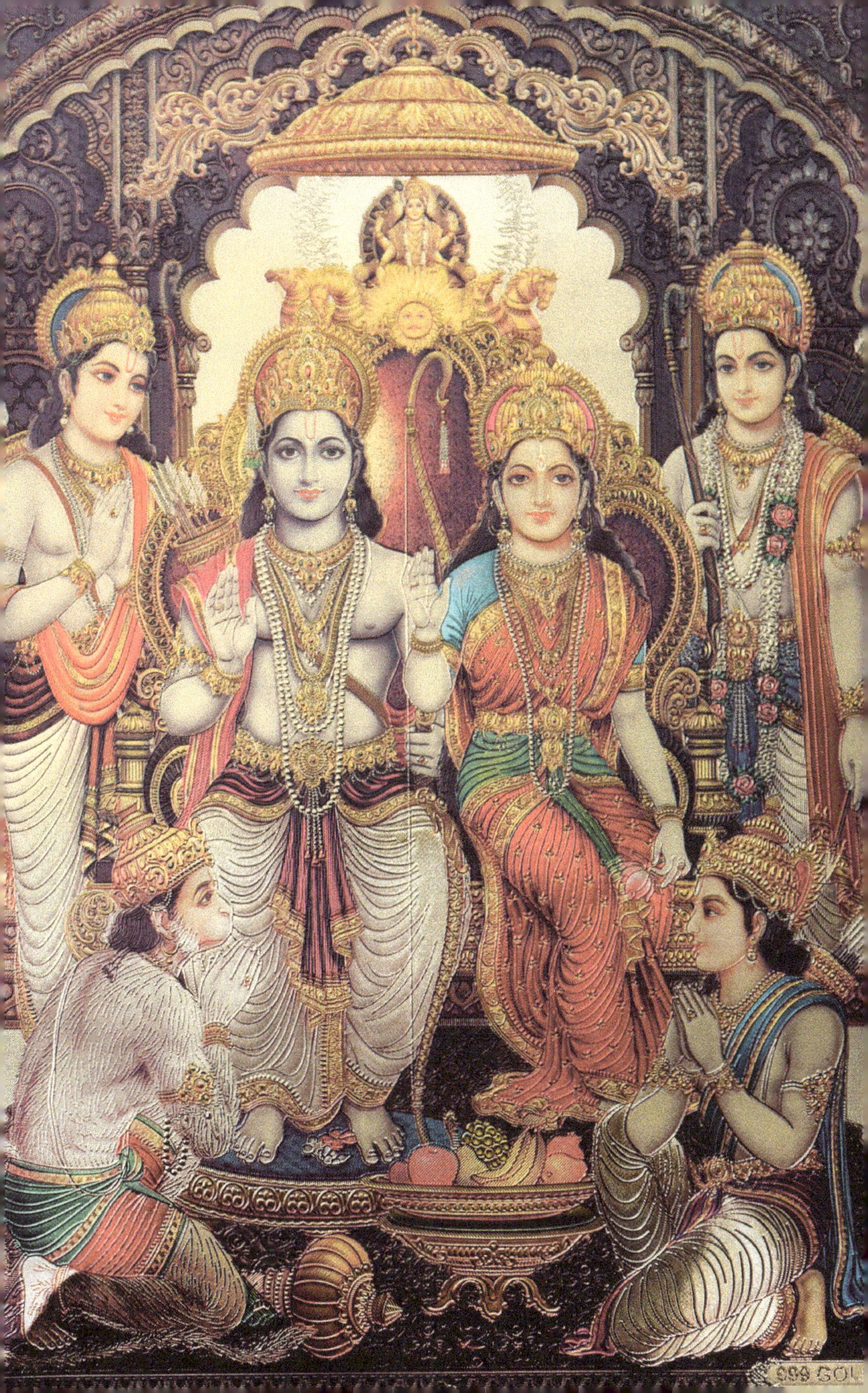

om sri dhanvantre namaha

Om Shree Don-von-trey Nahm-ah-ha

Om – Sacred sound
Sri – Reverence, auspiciousness
Dhanvantre – To Dhanvantari, the celestial physician
Namaha – I bow

Salutations to Lord Dhanvantari, the divine healer and source of Ayurveda.

Invoking the Celestial Physician, **Dhanvantre**, opens doors to the proper path in healing, including finding the right medical practitioners and cures. The Dhanvantre mantra is potent in several ways. It can bring spiritual healing into the body as well as direct the seeker to physicians and healers who can help with the issue. The appropriate healers and remedies often show up after chanting to Dhanvantre, and it can also evoke the healer's highest skills in serving the patient.

This mantra helps one become more intuitive about what the body needs to restore balance and can bring healing light and spiritual *prana* into the body, similar to the Ram mantra. While chanting, one can place their hands on the ailing area to invoke the celestial healer and bring divine life force and energetic balance. The hands often become warm or tingly as the palm chakras open, transmitting healing current.

In traditional households in southern India, women chant this mantra while preparing food to infuse it with healing vibrations believed to ward off disease. It is also recited to aid in the recovery of those who are sick or infirm.

I have used this mantra frequently when I've had health concerns. After about ten minutes of chanting with my hands on the afflicted area, I can feel a healing pulse flowing through them, and I continue until the body tension eases. While chanting, I often receive insights such as "it's your psoas – go see the chiropractor and acupuncturist" or "get some adrenal tonic – your adrenals are tapped!"

I recommended this mantra to a client recovering from Covid who wasn't improving after several weeks. During a virtual session we chanted together, and I received the message that she was suffering from excess spike protein residual from the virus. I suggested possible supplements but told her to keep chanting. The next day she reported her brain fog and drowsiness had cleared after chanting for several hours.

According to Namadeva, "this mantra can be chanted while concentrating upon any condition that you would like remedied or healed. Chant it at least 12,500 times, then be open to the manner in which healing will manifest. Remember that healing may be achieved according to traditional medicine or through other means. Be open-minded and do not hold expectations of how the healing will occur."*

* Thomas Ashley-Farrand, *Healing Mantras: Using Sound Affirmations for Personal Power, Creativity, and Healing* (New York: Ballantine Books, 1999), 113.

Om Hum Hanumate Namaha

Om Hum Hah-noo-mah-teh Nahm-ah-ha

Om – Sacred sound
Hum – *Bija* sound representing divine power, protection, and purification
Hanumate – To Hanuman, the great devotee of Lord Rama
Namaha – I bow

Salutations to Lord Hanuman, the embodiment of strength, devotion, and protection.

This mantra invokes the Vedic deity, Hanuman, for health, strength, and agility. It reinforces the conscious life principle with vigorous energy and can also clear blockages in the body, energy field, or lifestream. This mantra enhances *prana* which is considered the force that animates all living beings. It is the energy that flows through the body and sustains life, and is activated by breath. Chanting this mantra can palpably bring more energy into the body and make one feel vitalized. It can be used to feel better when one is sluggish or feeling down. It makes the life force conscious and then can be directed to where healing is needed.

My client used this mantra when she began to feel ill while traveling. Lucy had to wake up very early to catch a flight, and was feeling groggy and exhausted from sleep deficiency. She was getting a sore throat as well. To make it worse, when Lucy arrived at the airport gate, she saw her flight had been delayed for four hours. Her lack of sleep and early wake up time seemed in vain. She was awaiting a six hour flight from Boston to the West Coast when she decided to text me. In desperation she asked what mantra she should chant to feel better and not get sick during this long lag time. I told her to start chanting "Om Hum Hanumate Namaha," immediately and throughout her plane ride. Within five minutes of chanting it, the flight departure was moved up. Then she continued chanting and started to feel better and had a restorative sleep during the plane ride. She was energized and wide awake upon arrival. At baggage claim, her luggage showed up in record time, and an Uber arrived immediately. When she arrived at her hotel she was upgraded to a luxury suite! "Om Hum Hanumate Namaha," not only helped Lucy feel better, but she received added benefits of swiftness and an upgrade!

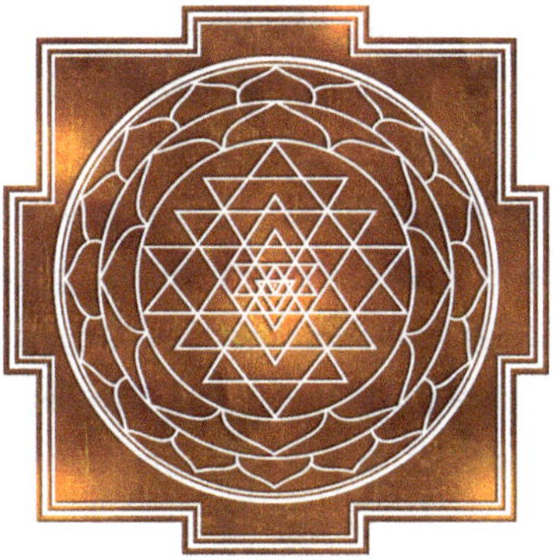

Om Tryam-bakam Yajamahe Sughandhim Pushti-vardanam Urvar-ukamiva Bandhanan Mrityor Mukshiya Mamritat

Om Try-um-bah-kum Ya-jahm-mah-hey Soo-gahn-dim Poosh-tee-vahr-dah-nahm Oor-vahr-oo-kumee-vah Bahn-dahn-ahn Mrit-your Mook-shee-yah Mahm-ree-taht

Om – Sacred sound
Tryambakam – The three-eyed one (a reference to Lord Shiva, whose third eye symbolizes inner vision and spiritual wisdom)
Yajamahe – We worship, honor, or adore
Sugandhim – The fragrant one; refers to divine qualities that are pleasing, uplifting, and pure
Pushtivardhanam – The one who nourishes and strengthens well-being and vitality
Urvarukamiva – Like a cucumber or ripened fruit (used as a metaphor for natural detachment)
Bandhanan – From bondage or attachment
Mrityor – From death
Mukshiya – May (you) liberate
Ma Amritat – Not from immortality; i.e., "Do not let me be separated from immortality"

Oh three-eyed Shiva who is fragrant, bless me with health and immortality, and sever me from the clutches of death, even as we separate a cucumber from its creeper.

This is a powerful Shiva Mantra known by several names, such as the Mritunjaya and **Markandeya** mantra. This mantra protects against "that which destroys death and disease." Namadeva viewed it as one of two most powerful mantras from the Vedic tradition. The other healing mantra he revered was the Apadamapa mantra of Rama (to be shared in a future book). The Markandeya mantra can be applied for any medical, emotional, or mental problem.

I find this is another mantra that is very fast acting and profound when chanting it and putting one's hands on the affected body area. Energy pulses through the hands very strongly when this is chanted. This mantra also troubleshoots where the problem is in the body, if the origin of pain, or affliction is not clear. When one chants this, the part of the body where the issue is stored may begin to ache or have weird pains or energy arise. If one keeps chanting, the energy can be cleared and aches or pains go away. But it is advised to go to a medical practitioner or healer to follow up with the health issue.

The Mrityunjaya Mantra
by Dr. Alexi Jardine Martel

The Maha Mrityunjaya Mantra, sometimes referred to as the Shiva Tryumbukum mantra, is one of the most powerful healing mantras in the Vedic tradition. The legendary story of Markandeya recounts the mantra's origin. As the legend goes,

Markandeya was a very pious child with a pure heart and a mystical bend. The boy was fiercely devoted to Shiva, the embodiment of universal consciousness. However, due to circumstances around his birth Markandeya was fated to die upon turning 16. On his 16th birthday, Yama, the god of death, came to collect Markandeya's soul. Feeling his imminent death, the boy cried out to Shiva in his devotion and spontaneously uttered the Tryumbukum mantra. Shiva answered the boy's prayer and stopped his aging permanently right before he would have turned 16, thus preventing his foretold death.

Markandeya is still remembered as an immortal sage said to wander the Himalayas to this day. His prayer to Lord Shiva became known as the Maha Mrityunjaya Mantra, which loosely translates to the Great Victory-over-Death Mantra. Invocation of this mantra is said to both protect and heal an individual from all manners of illnesses, injury, ill will, negative supernatural influences, and misfortune. The mantra also has the benefit of bestowing a profound peace of mind. It reaches deep into the depths of the chanter's psyche to help heal and protect them from their inner unconscious turmoil, which can sometimes manifest as neuroses or phobias. Essentially, the mantra helps to re-groove negative patterns of thoughts or feelings, whether they are conscious or unconscious. As a more day-to-day application, the mantra is very good at relieving feelings of anxiety or dread. People familiar with this mantra typically chant it before beginning a long journey, when faced with illness, or when one's environment makes them nervous.

I can personally vouch for this mantra's uplifting and soothing energy. It is a calming influence for me when times are tough. The Maha Mrityunjaya Mantra is a powerful emotional armor to call upon whenever I face uncertainty, fear, anxiety, dread, or any sort of emotional grunge. I invoke it before beginning road trips or going to an airport or even when daily traffic gets dicey. When I feel a possible illness coming on, I will chant this mantra as well as boost up on protective supplements like zinc, monolaurin, and multivitamins. The Shiva Tryumbukum mantra is an energetic equivalent to a good nutritious meal that effectively addresses a nutritional deficit that you didn't know you had but feel much better upon addressing. As your energetic body adjusts to higher energetic frequencies through chanting Sanskrit mantras and other evolutionary practices, certain mantras become a key ingredient in your "mantra mealtime." Much as your body might crave a workout when you're in an active physical phase, so too can you come to crave the energetic upliftment of certain mantras that resonate deeply with you. The Maha Mrityunjaya Mantra is one such mantra for me; I cannot recommend it highly enough.

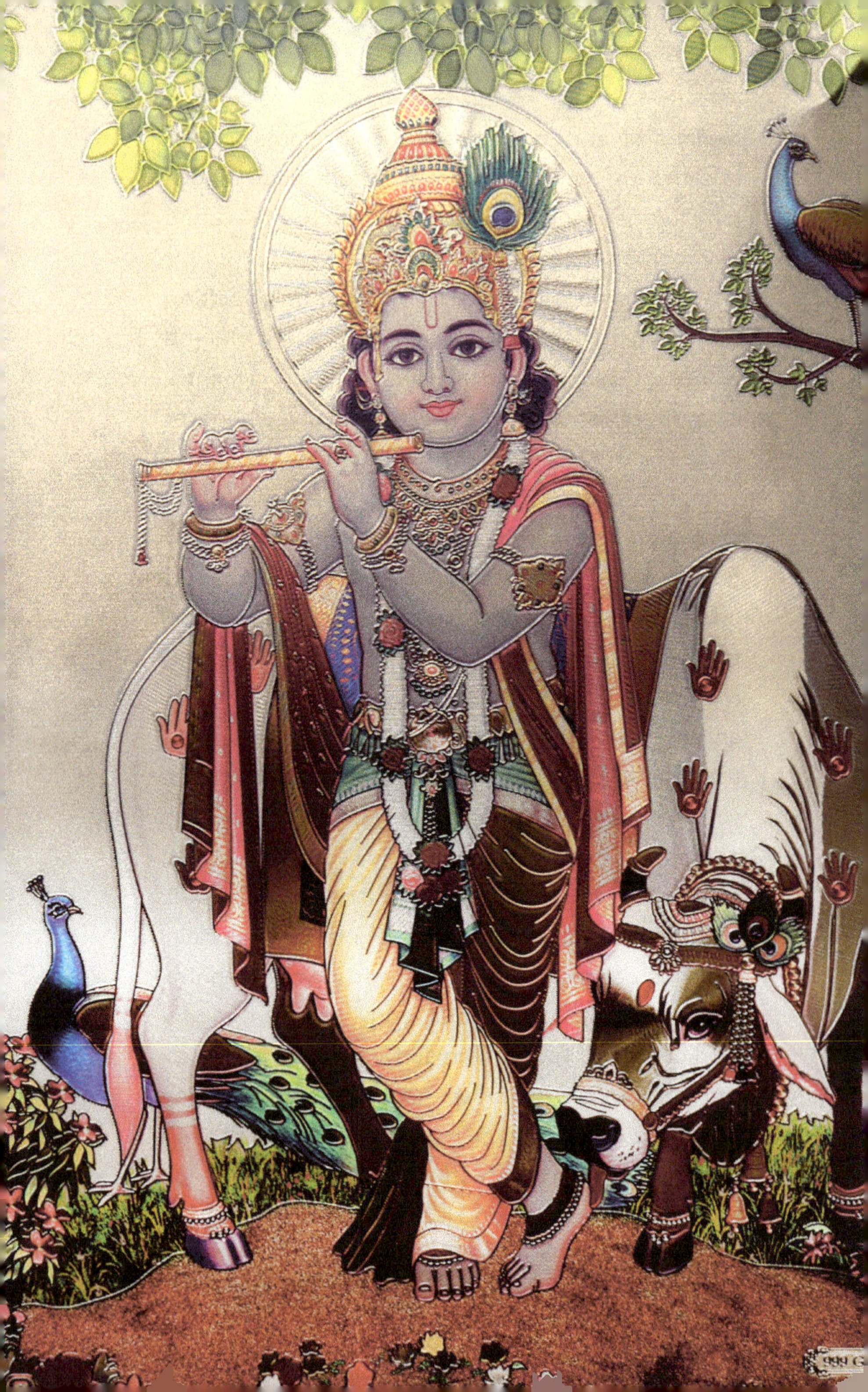

7

Mantras for Love and Relationships

The Krishna Principle

In the Hindu pantheon, Krishna is one of the most beloved and widely worshipped deities. He is considered the eighth incarnation of Vishnu, the preserver in the Hindu Trinity (Brahma the creator, Vishnu the preserver, and Shiva the transformer). However, to many devotees, Krishna is not merely an avatar but the Supreme Being himself, known as Svayam Bhagavan – the original, complete manifestation of God.

Krishna is often regarded as the most complete of Vishnu's avatars, embodying the fullest expression of Vishnu's divine energy. While all avatars of Vishnu – such as Rama and Narasimha – carry profound spiritual significance, Krishna is said to manifest the totality of divinity in human form. Like the other great incarnations, his earthly appearance is shrouded in spiritual mystery and cosmic purpose.

One of the most fascinating aspects of Krishna's life is the profound attraction he evoked, especially among women. According to ancient texts, 16,108 women are said to have fallen in love with him. This has long been a subject of mystical interpretation. Some spiritual teachers suggest that this love was not physical in nature, but rather a transmutation of human desire into the higher frequency of Divine Love. Others acknowledge the physical dimension but emphasize that, even so, the ultimate outcome was the same: the elevation of human love into a sublime, spiritual union with the Divine.

Krishna is the purest embodiment of *prema* – Divine Love in its most exalted and unconditional form. He does not merely represent love; he is love in motion, love made manifest. Through his eternal union with **Radha**, the Divine Feminine, the Radha-Krishna principle expresses the highest mystical truth: the union of the individual soul with the Supreme. Their love transcends physicality, pointing instead to a timeless and sacred path of inner devotion, where longing itself becomes a bridge to Divine union.

The sound of Krishna's flute is more than a melody – it is a vibrational call from the soul's original home. It draws beings irresistibly toward him, symbolizing the deep inner yearning each soul carries to return to Source. His **lilas**, or divine plays, are not simply mythic stories but ecstatic revelations of spiritual truth. They invite the seeker to move beyond mind and merge into the ecstatic rhythm of joy, surrender, and unity.

Krishna is not just a deity – he is a frequency, the radiant blueprint of the soul's innate bliss. To chant his name is to align with that frequency, to awaken and entrain the subtle body to the vibration of Divine Love. This sacred sound current stirs dormant devotion, rekindles remembrance of the Self, and reactivates the soul's original essence: joy, connection, and sacred belonging.

Love and money are pursuits that most people are seeking at some point in their life, (if not their entire life). Love falls under the category of *kama* in the Vedic *Purusharthas* (aims of life) while money is part of *artha*, the pursuit of material success, prosperity, and security. *Kama* means love in Sanskrit, and Kamala is the goddess of Love, a manifestation of Lakshmi.

Prema is Divine Love; *bhakti* is another Sanskrit word associated with love, but this refers to a devotional type of love. *Bhakti* is love in its purest form, directed toward God or the Divine in a personal or impersonal form. It may be expressed as reverence, yearning, gratitude, or joyful praise, which can be chanted and sung. The *bhakta* (devotee) loves God not for any personal gain, liberation, or fulfillment, but surrenders to the energy of love. The devotee no longer distinguishes between self and Divine. All that remains is a boundless longing, surrender, and joy in the Beloved's presence.

This chapter includes mantras for personal love, Divine Love, and self love. When clients come to see me, love and relationships are often at the top of their list of concerns – topics they most frequently ask me to explore astrologically and energetically during our sessions. These concerns may be because they have ended a relationship and feel ready to find a new one, or they have realized they have a particular pattern of attracting the wrong type of person. Another common situation people want help with is to improve an existing relationship whether it is burgeoning one or a marriage at various stages. The mantras I share in this chapter are the ones I most frequently prescribe for those looking for love and relationships. This includes those who want to attract a new relationship, heal an existing relationship, feel more self-love, and connect with Divine Love.

Mantras can amplify your natural magnetism, aligning your energy with what resonates in your life – whether it's a new job, a romantic partner, or any opportunity that matches your elevated vibration. As we have discussed earlier in the book, mantras work by refining and elevating your inner vibration, bringing you into greater harmony with the subtle energies of the universe. As your energetic frequency aligns with your true intentions, you naturally begin to attract experiences, relationships, and opportunities – such as meaningful work or a compatible partner – that reflect this higher state of being. Mantras can raise your vibration to help you meet your match again in another person or energetically with what it is that you desire to bring in, which can also be health and wealth. When we are trying to bring more love into our life, the best place to start is with creating more self-love. If one loves themselves or feels confident, that is putting a higher frequency out into the world than one who is self-loathing, depressed, or a naysayer. The love mantras here will enhance the energies of self-love, but also cultivate feelings of confident self-love and empowerment. It's so much more than just attracting a mate. It's allowing you to heal yourself, going into the psyche and clearing blocks or lack of confidence and other self-defeating or self-sabotaging behaviors and thoughts. Sanskrit mantras, by the nature of their vibrations, will help weed out psychological complexes, blockages, issues, and even patterns that you may not be aware of consciously which interfere with attracting an appropriate relationship.

It is advised to never chant to manipulate someone with mantras or cast love spells. The karmic rebound on whoever does so can be very fast in delivering negative outcomes. *Vashikarana* mantras are a type of mantra that reek of manipulation and can hold the energy of black magic. They are used with the intent to attract, influence, or gain control over someone, typically in the context of love, relationships, or persuasion. It is never a good idea to cultivate that type of bad karma. In relationships, it's important not to create karmic entanglements through actions rooted in attachment, manipulation, or harm.

It is important not to become overly fixated on another person when pursuing a relationship. Such obsession breeds attachment and desire – qualities that stand in direct opposition to the soul's liberation, which is the deeper aim of mantra practice. Clinging to a specific outcome or individual lowers your energetic vibration and can lead to emotional instability.

In my experience, I've observed several female clients become deeply infatuated with certain men – often to the extent of constructing imagined relationships, despite minimal or no reciprocation from the other side. This kind of fixation is not only unhealthy, but it also tends to repel the very person they seek, as the intensity of their emotional projection creates an unspoken pressure that others can sense and instinctively pull away from.

When chanting for love, center yourself in your own heart and offer your intentions to the Divine. Surrender your desire to be fulfilled not by personal will, but by divine grace – unfolding in perfect timing, for the highest and holiest good of all souls involved.

As I tell my clients and friends, "who needs dating apps when we have Sanskrit mantras for love!"

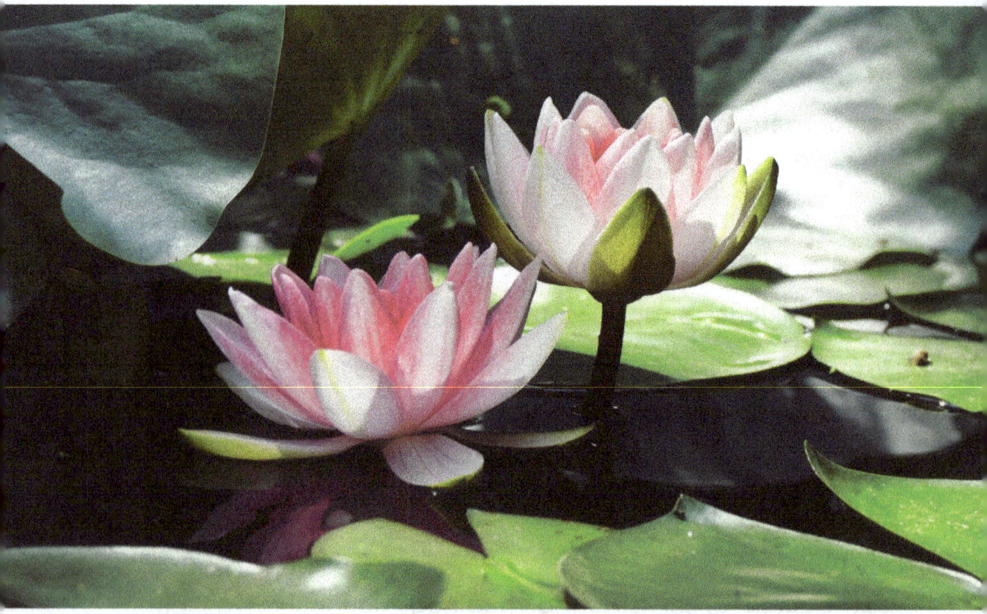

om klim krishnaya namaha

Om Kleem Krish-nah-yah Nahm-ah-ha

Om – Sacred sound
Klim – Seed sound for attraction and devotion (often associated with Krishna or the Divine Feminine)
Krishnaya – To Krishna, the divine incarnation of Vishnu
Namaha – I bow

Salutations to Krishna, the embodiment of divine love, joy, and devotion.

This mantra weaves together Klim, the seed sound of attraction, with the Krishna principle – the embodiment of Divine Love and the cosmic lover. It can be used to awaken and enhance love in all its forms – whether romantic, devotional, or self-directed.

By invoking the vibrant, heart-opening energy of Krishna, this mantra draws love into your life with grace and joy. For those seeking a male partner, Krishna often brings forth a connection that is playful, affectionate, and deeply heart-centered – mirroring His own qualities as the blissful beloved of the soul. This mantra can awaken devotion in the heart and cultivate more self-love as well as enhance one's connection to their Divine Source.

I recommended this mantra to a client who had recently gone through a difficult divorce which went on for several painful years and she hadn't been in a romantic relationship for quite some time. She was ready to open her heart again. Alongside that, I suggested she chant "Om Namah Shivaya" to invite positive and benevolent male energy, as her experience had left her wary and cautious about men.

The mantras worked quickly – within just a month, she attracted not one, but two very different men. One was more Krishna-like: charming, romantic, and attentive, wooing her with concerts, dinners, and romantic getaways. The other was an intense, no-nonsense attorney with a commanding presence – more Shiva-like, serious and brooding.

The takeaway? Mantras can work double time, bringing powerful energies into your life in unexpected ways. Why is it that women tend to go after the bad boy first, before realizing it was Krishna all along?

Postscript: The Shiva-like man was her boyfriend for a year and then he moved away. Though deep and intense, his moody nature made the relationship challenging. After he left, she began dating the Krishna-like man from before, and that relationship blossomed and lasted for many years.

om radha krishnaya namaha

Om Rad-hah Krish-nah-yah Nahm-ah-ha

Om – Sacred sound
Radha – Divine consort of Krishna, symbol of pure love and devotion
Krishnaya – To Krishna, the divine lover and avatar of Vishnu
Namaha – I bow

Salutations to Radha and Krishna, the embodiment of divine love and bliss.

This mantra combines the divine feminine principle of love, Radha, with Krishna, the divine masculine expression of love and devotion, Radha represents total surrender, pure longing and union beyond union. She loves Krishna because he is love itself, and she isn't necessarily looking for his reciprocity. In some traditions, Radha's love is seen as greater than Krishna himself, because it embodies the Supreme Power of devotion.

This mantra activates the feminine energy *shakti* through Radha, and masculine consciousness symbolized by Krishna. Their union is symbolic of inner spiritual balance and harmony.

This mantra opens the heart center, allowing you to feel and give love more freely – both human and divine. Chanting it can connect one to *bhakti*, devotional love, and melts the ego. It is considered one of the best mantras for healing a relationship. It can bring more harmony, understanding, and love into romantic and emotional relationships. It can attract spiritually aligned partners. "Om Radha Krishnaya Namaha" may heal the heart if a relationship ends or there is separation from the beloved.

I prescribed this mantra to a client who discovered her husband was cheating on her with another woman. He admitted he had been having an affair for a few months. She was so sad that he had strayed, but didn't necessarily want to end the marriage. She had suggested he move out of their house until she decided what she wanted to do. I suggested she chant the mantra while feeling love in her heart for herself and remaining neutral about how to proceed. She experienced a calmness and soothing energy from chanting the mantra. She told me she felt as if she was becoming the embodiment of love. Her friends commented that she was glowing, and thought she had found another man to get even with her husband. She told them she was discovering the true meaning of self love and she felt guided by a higher power of love. She was flooded with memories from when she first dated her husband, and their early years of marriage when they were very much in love and shared many uplifting activities. She sent love to her younger self while chanting the mantra. She remembered the fun they had together and how alive she felt. Within a few weeks, her husband was begging to move back home and admitting that he had made a big mistake. He had broken it off with the other woman, who then became obsessive, and was stalking him. He had to get a restraining order on her. He realized he had opened a Pandora's box by having an affair, and that the grass was not greener away from home. My client forgave him, on a trial basis, but insisted they do activities like hiking and tennis which they did when their relationship was new. They started taking weekend trips staying at resorts in Vermont and Maine, and rekindled their love of hiking and doing other activities together. They are still going strong ten years later.

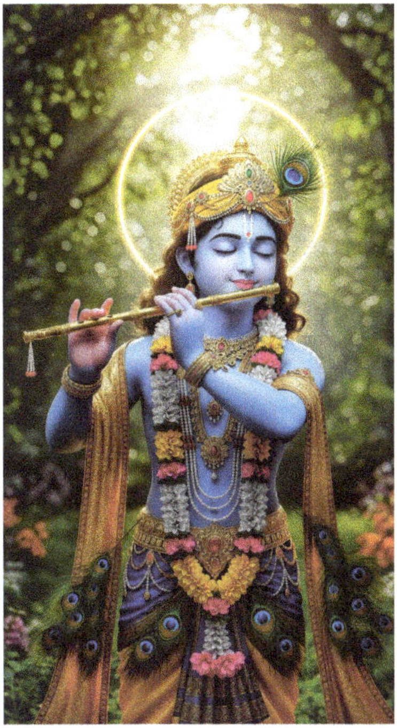

Om Kamala-Yei Namaha

Om Kah-mah-lah-yei Nahm-ah-ha

Om – Sacred sound
Kamala – Lotus, also a name for Goddess Lakshmi
Yei – Feminine dative ending (to the goddess)
Namaha – I bow

**Salutations to the lotus goddess Kamala,
the radiant aspect of Lakshmi.**

This is a very easy love mantra to chant and feels very good when chanting. It can also bestow more self-love, as well as attracting a partner or transforming an existing relationship.

When chanting for love, turn inward and rest in the sanctuary of your heart. Offer your longing to Kamala, the embodiment of Divine Love and devotion. Surrender your desire at her lotus feet, trusting that she will fulfill it under her grace, in the highest and most harmonious way – for the upliftment of all hearts involved. Let your chant be not a plea, but a prayer of love, offered in surrender and faith.

Chanting this mantra invokes the energy of Kamala who embodies softness, elegance, and divine worth. Her presence nurtures your sense of inner beauty, increasing self-respect, self-love, and magnetism. When you love yourself deeply and gracefully, you naturally attract love in return. Chanting her name can help draw loving, supportive, and respectful partners into your life – especially relationships that are aligned with *dharma* and inner growth.

This mantra is chanted to attract a relationship or partner (female or male). It is very effective for improving an existing relationship, especially during its initial phases or in the onset. Chanting to Kamala can also bring harmony to a rocky relationship if it is meant to be in one's best interest. Kamala's energy is soothing and nourishing. If you've been through heartbreak, emotional neglect, or toxic relationships, this mantra can help repair the emotional body, gently restoring trust in love and allowing your heart to bloom again.

Beyond romantic love, this mantra elevates your heart toward Divine Love – the kind of love that is unconditional, surrendered, and radiant. It helps you connect to love as a sacred force, not just an emotion.

I have recommended this mantra to several clients who attracted relationships shortly after chanting this mantra. Jennifer, a 46-year-old pharmaceutical sales representative, had come to see me for a reading. She wanted me to look at her astrological chart to see if there was anything in it that blocked her finding love. She was disappointed with a series of men she had met through online dating, who all ended up being "duds." She hadn't been in a serious relationship for five years. She joked that she was ready to "get thee to a nunnery." I asked her if she felt she was willing to give it another chance, but not use the dating apps. I also asked her if she was ready to go beyond dating and actually have a relationship. She answered with a resounding "Yes!" I told her she would have to be committed to chanting a Sanskrit mantra 108 times a day minimally. I asked her if she wanted one, two, or three mantras. She was honest and said she could only see herself chanting one Sanskrit mantra a day, and the easier to say the better. So I prescribed "Om Kamalayei Namaha." I also suggested she purchase a rose quartz mala to dedicate to chanting this mantra, and told her where to find one. She left me and purchased the rose quartz mala. Rose quartz is a crystal that is recommended as a love stone. She started chanting it immediately, and texted me the next day that she felt really good when chanting it, and had already chanted five malas of it within 24 hours. The next day she texted me that felt that some heaviness around her heart had been released and she felt lighter. On the third day, she attended a music concert that night at an outdoor venue. She met a man and he bought her a drink and they danced. He took her phone number, and called her the next day. They went out that weekend. She had only been chanting the mantra a week and went on her first date with him. They liked the same type of music and appreciated each others sense of humor. The following weekend they went to a concert. They continued dating and became exclusive with each other after three months. Jennifer kept chanting, "Om Kamalayei Namaha." Flash forward a year later and they became engaged.

sat patim dehi paramesh-waraya

Saht Pah-teem Day-hee Pah-rahm-esh-wah-rah-ya

Om – Sacred sound
Sat – True, righteous, noble, or virtuous
Patim – Husband or life partner
Dehi – Grant me, bestow upon me
Parameshwara – O Supreme Lord / Supreme Divine Being

Please give me a man of truth who embodies the perfect masculine attributes.

Parameshwara is a name for the masculine divinity, Shiva. This mantra is a prayer to Shiva or the "Supreme Lord, Parameshwara," asking for a virtuous husband.

This mantra is traditionally used in the context of marriage, particularly by unmarried women seeking a good life partner. It's important to chant with sincerity, clarity of purpose, and devotion.

I have an amazing story of a client who chanted the "Sat Patim Dehi Parameshwara" mantra to attract a spiritual husband. Things aligned in her life for the energy of this mantra to flow in and bring her a successful outcome. Sally was a hard-working 29-year-old client who came to me because she wanted to attract love, specifically a committed relationship. Her advertising job was demanding and she traveled extensively. She told me she had been so focused on getting ahead in her job and financially, that the relationship part of her life had been on the back burner. She wanted a man who was in the same phase of life as she was, had a good job, was never married and with no children. I asked her if she was seriously ready for marriage and would create space in her life for a man and children eventually.

I told Sally that she was in her Saturn Return astrologically, which is a time of endings and beginnings. The first Saturn Return occurs between 28-30 years old and it is a good time to restructure one's life for the next 29 years. The deity that rules Saturn in Vedic astrology is Shiva, and "Sat Patim Dehi Parameshwara" is asking Shiva to bring in a spiritual husband. She said, "Let's go!" I also suggested she get a **rudraksha** mala to chant this mantra on exclusively. The rudraksha seed is sacred to Shiva. I also recommended the feng shui remedy of making space in her closet and bedroom for the incoming partner. I gave her the exercise of visualizing herself doing some of her favorite activities with the man. I told her don't focus on his face or body, but just see him as a pillar of light, across the tennis court from you or hiking next to you. Shiva is often invoked as a pillar of light. She was excited to begin that visualization and then make time every morning to chant the mantra. I also told her to chant a mala of "Om Gum Ganapatayei Namaha" to initiate her Sat Patim Dehi sadhana, and to start chanting it on a Saturday (Shiva's day).

Sally was a fast study as she followed my recommendations and began chanting the next day which was a Saturday. Some days she would chant more than one mala. I told her it was important to do a mantra discipline with this mantra by chanting at least one mala a day for a minimum of 40 days in a row. She had to travel to London for work several weeks later (35 days into her mantra discipline). I told her to keep chanting the mantra every day even when you are traveling. On the 40th day of the discipline she was in London, and arose very early to chant "Sat Patim Dehi Parameshwara," before flying home. She had flown Business Class on the way there but had upgraded herself to First Class for the flight home. She sat in the First Class aisle seat, and it seemed as if the seat next to her was going to be empty, until an attractive man rushed onto the plane and sat in the seat next to her. He said in his fluster, "I'm sorry I'm late," as if he was her husband or boyfriend. She thought was weird he said it to her, a total stranger. They ended up talking (and flirting) for most of the flight and realized they knew some of the same people in Boston. He asked for her phone number, and if she would want to meet up with him in Boston. They started dating and realized they had the same life goals, he was a few years older than her. By a year after the plane encounter, they were engaged and then married. They now have two young children and live in a suburb of Boston, happily ever after.

aham prema

Ah-hahm Preh-mah

Aham – I am
Prema – Divine love

I am divine love.

This is a simple yet powerful affirmation mantra for embodying unconditional love and spiritual unity. This mantra helps us realize that love resides within oneself. It is a teaching of yogic traditions that our essence is love, consciousness, and divinity. It is a simple heart mantra that brings self love, Divine Love, and can attract love from outside oneself.

This mantra can be used to feel the expansion of the heart chakra. It cultivates self-love and self-worth. It can be chanted to cultivate self-awareness, compassion, and inner peace. It will help you to love all parts of yourself, the good, bad, and ugly. One can chant this mantra to heal the younger self, the inner child, the inner teenager or to send love to the future self. This mantra can help you experience a sense of Divine Love – a presence beyond yourself that embraces you with unconditional affection. One can cultivate a connection with something greater than yourself in a loving way. By chanting this mantra one can vibrate or resonate in a tender hearted way and feel compassion towards all sentient beings. It also gives a radiance or glow which may attract people or good outcomes.

As a yoga and metaphysical workshop teacher, I guide the class to chant "Aham Prema" at the beginning or end of class or workshop so they can experience an open-hearted practice and send love to their body. I have participants put their left hand on their heart and their right hand on top of the left and chant. The energy is palpable in their hands and heart. It is a transformational experience. Spontaneous tears flow from the eyes, which we call "Bhakti tears," as a result of devotional love. I have the group chant it minimally 27 times which is enough to feel a powerful surge. When we chant a full mala of 108 repetition, people are blissed out. It is short and easy to chant and people take to it immediately. No one wants to leave the group energy at the end. Everyone is sitting or lying down in their personal and collective cocoon of love.

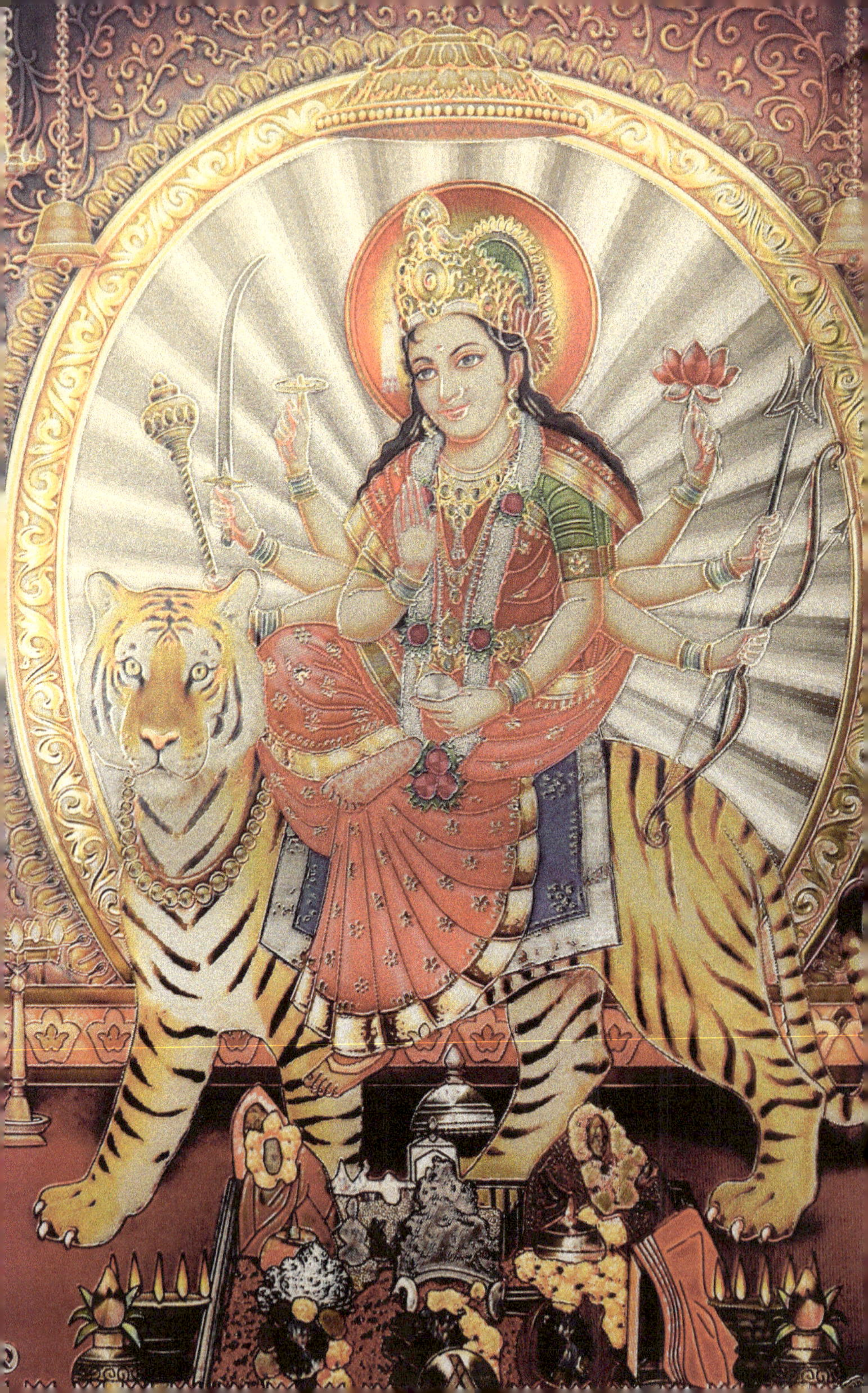

8

Mantras for Protection

The Durga Principle: The Radiant Protectress

Durga is the Divine Mother in her most protective form – both fierce and beautiful, wrathful and compassionate. She rides a lion or tiger, symbolic of her mastery over power and instinct, her serene yet commanding presence radiating supreme sovereignty. With a luminous face and many arms bearing weapons of light, Durga is the embodiment of fierce compassion – the force that defends truth, dissolves illusion, and shields the soul on its path to liberation.

To the sincere seeker of Truth, she is a benevolent guardian, a liberator from ignorance, negativity, and all that binds the spirit. Her weapons are not for the innocent – they are for their defense. She comes not to punish, but to protect, standing firm between the soul and any force that would cause harm. Her radiant smile soothes the heart of the devotee, whispering the timeless assurance that divine protection is always near.

Yet to the arrogant, the unjust, and the forces of oppression, she appears as a fearsome power – an unrelenting force of divine justice. Her eyes blaze with truth, her weapons flash with righteous purpose, and the lion beneath her feet coils with readiness. To such energies, she is a mirror of reckoning, awakening transformation through shock, fire, and dissolution.

Durga is most revered in those moments of life that demand unwavering strength and deep discernment – when devotion must be fortified by inner power, and love must be anchored in truth. She calls forth the spiritual warrior within, the part of us that refuses to be defeated by darkness.

For those drawn to the Mother aspect of the Divine – the nurturing yet potent feminine – Durga is a profoundly resonant presence. She is the Cosmic Mother who fiercely loves, fiercely protects, and fiercely liberates. In her embrace, one finds the courage to rise, the clarity to see, and the strength to walk the path of truth without fear.

In recent decades, the internet has become saturated with techniques and tools promising to accelerate spiritual growth – methods to open the third eye, awaken kundalini, enhance psychic abilities, and more. While these offerings can be genuinely helpful, they also cater to a subtle impulse of the ego: the desire to appear more spiritual, more awakened, or more powerful than others – a kind of spiritual one-upmanship that often circulates in New Age and modern yogic circles.

Amid the abundance of "how-to-be-more-spiritual" content, one critical element is often overlooked: the necessity of discernment. Rarely do these platforms emphasize the importance of spiritual discrimination – of knowing what is appropriate for one's path, timing, and energetic integrity. Even fewer address the essential need for energetic protection, especially when engaging with unfamiliar practices or altered states of consciousness.

In the pursuit of higher states, wisdom must walk hand in hand with aspiration. Without discernment, the seeker becomes vulnerable – not only to energetic confusion, but to spiritual bypassing and subtle forms of self-deception. True evolution demands not just access to tools, but the inner clarity to know which ones to use – and when to walk away.

Spiritual protection has long been regarded as essential within authentic Eastern traditions and esoteric lineages. Teachings from Tibetan Buddhism, Tantric paths, and other ancient systems take the unseen realms seriously, offering precise methods for shielding the practitioner from harmful energies and disturbances encountered on the path of awakening. These systems recognize that as one opens to subtler dimensions, one also becomes more sensitive – and therefore more vulnerable – to energetic interference.

In contrast, spiritual protection in the West often appears in more symbolic or superficial forms – such as wearing an "evil eye" talisman, protective jewelry, or other charms believed to ward off negative influences. Folk traditions such as Greek, Italian, Romani (Gypsy), and Wiccan practices may employ spells to dispel unwanted energies or to protect against harm. Yet spellwork itself carries its own karmic weight and complexities. Without deep wisdom and ethical grounding, such practices can unintentionally entangle the practitioner in the very forces they seek to avoid, sometimes even attracting what they hope to repel.

Within Christian and other Abrahamic traditions, rituals such as exorcisms serve a similar purpose – intended to cast out malevolent entities or purify spaces afflicted by spiritual darkness. Though often dramatized, these rites point to a long-standing understanding that unseen energies can influence human consciousness and behavior.

Today, the need for energetic protection extends beyond the esoteric or religious realm. In an age where emotional and psychological toxins are routinely unleashed through digital channels – especially on political and social media platforms – many find themselves energetically drained, overwhelmed, or destabilized by the projections and hostility of others. The negativity of the collective ego, amplified through polarized discourse, can infiltrate the mind and erode one's inner clarity.

Yet perhaps the greatest threat does not come from the outside. One's own unexamined ego – particularly its shadow aspects – can be the most persistent saboteur. Internalized fear, judgment, envy, and resentment form gateways through which negative energies can take root. Thus, the path of spiritual protection is not only about shielding from outer forces, but also about becoming aware of – and transmuting – the inner tendencies that leave us open to harm.

True protection arises from clarity, integrity, and deep alignment with one's higher Self. As the ancients knew, it is not merely a defense, but a way of walking in the world with awakened presence and unshakable sovereignty.

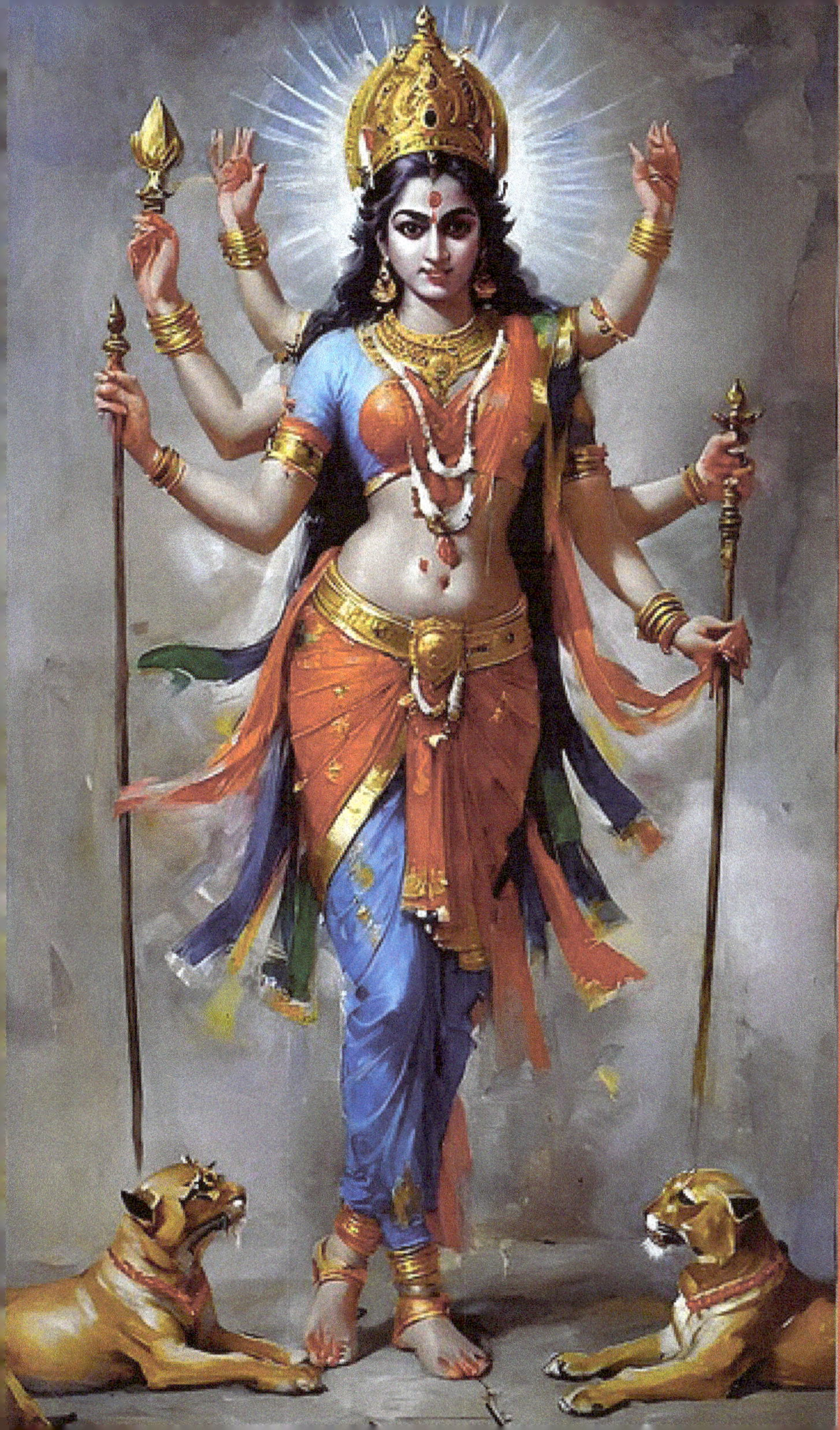

om shakti ganapatayei namaha

Om Shak-tee Ga-na-pa-ta-yei Nahm-ah-ha

Om – Sacred sound
Shakti – Divine feminine power
Ganapatayei – To Ganesha
Namaha – I bow

Salutations to Ganesha in his form united with divine feminine power – the remover of obstacles energized by Shakti.

This mantra invokes Shakti to remove obstacles. According to Sadguru Sant Keshavadas in *Lord Ganesha*, the mantra can be used specifically, "to cast away evil spirits from a haunted house or from the body or mind of a person."* He suggests that one meditates on the brown color of Ganesha when chanting it.

As in all Ganesha mantras it will remove obstacles, but also invokes Shakti, the divine feminine force or inner strength. It can be chanted at the beginning of one or more protective mantras. It invokes Ganapati for removal of blockages and clarity. "Om Shakti Ganapatayei Namaha" protects from negative people, entities, or places. It will dispel negativity, hatred, inner or outer enemies, and the demonic egos of self or others. It can also help one to seek

* Sadguru Sant Keshavadas, *Lord Ganesha* (Vishwa Dharma Publications, 1988), 27.

empowerment and divine guidance. It can be used as a space clearing mantra in a home or any environment.

In my capacity as a healer and Reverend in Sanskrit mantras, I am frequently hired to come and "clear" and/or bless houses and businesses. I reside in an earlier established, historic area of Massachusetts so there are many older homes and buildings. Two towns close by, Plymouth and Duxbury, Massachusetts, are widely recognized for their fair share of "haunted houses," and eerie areas. When I do a house clearing, I perform special prayers and other practices, including Sanskrit mantras. When chanting mantras to clear I always invoke Ganesha first. I then chant "Om Shakti Ganapatayei Namaha," and other Ganesha mantras for the first round of clearing while burning sage or spritzing holy water. I have witnessed some paranormal activity, including things flying off tables or shelves and things breaking, or hearing high pitched frequencies, and smelling weird scents, and other phenomena. I continue chanting and doing the process of clearing the space, and then if it gets more intense I will follow with other intense clearing mantras, like "Om Namo Bhagavate Rudraya" or the Narasimha mantra below. The paranormal activity tends to cease after about 20-30 minutes and I have witnessed the negative energies and entities leaving out of open windows and doors with whishing like sounds or with other noises. This mantra is also effective to chant to clear hotel rooms and rental properties.

om namo bhagavate rudraya

Om Nah-mo Bhah-gah-vah-teh Rud-rah-yah

Om – Sacred sound
Namo – Salutations
Bhagavate – To the divine, the Lord
Rudraya – To Rudra (a fierce form of Shiva)

Salutations to the divine Rudra, fierce and transformative form of Lord Shiva.

This mantra invokes a fierce manifestation of Shiva, in the form of Rudra, for protection and to cast away demons, negativity and bad energies. Rudra destroys ego, ignorance, and inner impurities. He clears away obstacles through fierce compassion and paves the way for transformation and spiritual rebirth. Chanting this mantra invokes divine protection, purifies the heart and mind, and brings inner strength during times of turmoil or transition. It is a mantra of surrendering to divine will, by releasing ego and need for control.

This powerful mantra can be chanted in times of adversity, especially when facing challenges that feel overwhelming or insurmountable.

It can be used to free attachments, entities, internal or outer enemies, and negative energies. Chanting to Rudra helps release karmic patterns, and offers strength, courage, and clarity when going through loss, grief, or major life changes. This mantra invokes Rudra's energy for protection from harm, both seen and unseen. It is very grounding as well as protective, and centers the practitioner in truth and spiritual power. This mantras dissolves ego and aligns with higher consciousness while deepening the connection to the universal and transcendent nature of Shiva.

I recommended the mantra "Om Namo Bhagavate Rudraya" to my client Karen, who was facing an unresolved $500,000 debt from her former marriage after her ex-husband died without a will. For two years, she endured relentless bank notices and conflicting legal advice, leaving her anxious and sleepless.

One Friday, she found a demand notice taped to her front door and called me in tears. In an emergency session, I suggested the Rudra mantra – not for finances, but because Rudra, a form of Shiva, rules over death and transformation. Karen began chanting nonstop. The very next day which was a Saturday, she miraculously got in to see a lawyer, who sent an email to the bank's attorney. She had to wait over the weekend while the situation was still unresolved. She chanted every waking hour. On Monday, her attorney called the bank's attorney, and after a discussion and clarification of the issues the pending debt was dismissed due to a legal loophole. Karen was overwhelmed with relief and gratitude.

Om Dum Durgayei Namaha

Om Doom Door-gah-yei Nahm-ah-ha

Om – Sacred sound
Dum – *Bija* mantra of protection and strength (linked to Durga)
Durgayei – To Goddess Durga
Namaha – I bow

**Salutations to Goddess Durga,
fierce protector and destroyer of evil.**

This is an easy mantra to chant which invokes Goddess Durga for protection from evil, danger, and negative forces. It can bestow inner strength and courage during challenging times. Durga can also help remove difficult or oppressive obstacles emotionally, spiritually, and physically. This mantra invokes Shakti, divine feminine empowerment. This can be chanted for protection for self or a loved one who is faced with a difficult situation. This is the mantra to chant at Lunar Eclipses to protect from any malefic energies that are being stirred up.

This is one of the mantras I prescribe frequently to clients, in addition to "Om Gum Ganapatayei Namaha." The reason is that everyone can use more protection and removal of obstacles. Vedic Astrologers recommend to chant Ganesha and Durga mantras at eclipses to mitigate negative influences.

I always recommend this mantra for parents to chant for the safety and well-being of their children (at any age). Even when children have left the home, this is a powerful mantra to invoke their protection.

Over the years, many women navigating divorce have come to me for guidance – both as an astrologer and therapist. One of the first things I recommend is chanting the mantra "Om Dum Durgayei Namaha" to invoke protection for themselves and their children during this emotionally charged time.

Divorce is often a difficult and contentious process. The energetic tension can be palpable, and children – sensitive to the emotional atmosphere – frequently absorb that stress, sometimes suffering in ways that are not immediately visible. Durga protects the psyche and welfare of those going through divorce, sometimes minimizing the damage financially and mentally. Her mantra creates a protective field, and I've seen it help alleviate emotional, psychological, and even financial harm.

Relationships are always karmic in nature, and during divorce, unresolved karmic threads are often being unraveled. Things may not go as expected because karmic debts are coming due. Chanting the Durga mantra can help stabilize the process and soften the karmic impact, offering strength, clarity, and protection along the way.

om eim hrim klim chamundayei vicche namaha

Om I'm Hreem Kleem Cha-mun-da-yay
Vich-chay Nahm-ah-ha

Om – Sacred sound
Eim – Wisdom (Saraswati)
Hrim – Divine power (Shakti)
Klim – Attraction, love (Krishna/Shakti)
Chamundayei – To Chamunda (a fierce form of the Goddess who defeats demons)
Vicche – Realization, awakening (often used in Tantric mantras to cut illusion)
Namaha – I bow

Salutations to Goddess Chamunda, who grants wisdom, power, and divine realization.

I bow to the Supreme Goddess Chamunda, an aspect of Goddess Durga, who embodies wisdom, strength, and attraction; may she cut through all illusions and obstacles. This mantra invokes the fierce and formidable aspect of the Divine Feminine for proactive protection and the destruction of negative forces or entities. This is a Tantric mantra because it uses seed sounds, "om, eim, hrim, klim," which carry a strong potency.

This mantra can be chanted to improve one's sense of comfort in any situation. It gives empowerment, preservation, protection, and creates a *kavacha* (spiritual armor for defense and safety, either physically, spiritually, or symbolically).

It can cut through negativity and fear. It bestows victory (*vicche*) over inner and outer enemies. Namadeva attributed this mantra to produce feelings of self-confidence, especially in women.

I gave this mantra to a young woman named Julia, who was preparing for a long drive from Massachusetts back to her college in Pennsylvania after winter break. She felt anxious about the weather, even though the forecast along her route was clear – no storms or snow expected.

To ease her concerns, I first recommended chanting Ganesha mantras to remove any obstacles from her path. Then I encouraged her to focus on the powerful invocation "Om Eim Hrim Klim Chamundayei Vicche Namaha" during the drive.

She had a recording of me chanting it on her phone, but I urged her to chant it aloud herself – so the vibration would come directly from her own voice and breath, activating its protective energy from within.

She texted me the next day to let me know she had arrived safely, but if it wasn't for the mantra she may not have made it. She said something miraculous had occurred and she wanted to tell me. Julia began chanting as soon as she hit the highway. Driving was swift with minimal traffic; the first few hours flew by, she was making good time. Then she hit a snow squall on the highway that came out of nowhere which made visibility impossible. She didn't want to pull over because she was afraid of being hit by trucks or other cars sliding into her. She saw cars that had slid off the highway. She felt an invisible protection surrounding her with a bubble of light and heard a voice say, "Keep driving!" She was white knuckling it for about 30 minutes, and then started chanting loudly. All of a sudden it was as if the sun came out and was shining down showing her the highway in front of her. Behind her it was dark and stormy, and she couldn't see the cars behind her or in the lane next to her. This mystical spotlight led her through the storm and all of a sudden it cleared up, and she saw her exit coming up. She did the math and it didn't make sense that she had made the six hour trip in half the time. She made it back to her campus apartment, and her roommate was surprised to see Julia. She said she didn't expect to see her for several more hours based on the text Julia had sent her at the onset of her trip. The roommate also asked Julia which route she had taken because of the bad storm which had hit, which closed down the main highway because of accidents. Julia was shocked, and told her that was the road she had just traveled on. They both just stared at each other in disbelief as something supernatural had occurred during Julia's drive. Julia realized it was the mantra "Om Eim Hrim Klim Chahmundayei Vicche Namaha" protecting her in an otherworldly way during the hazardous driving experience.

narasimha ta va da so hum

Nah-rah-seem-hah Tah Vah Dah So Hum

Narasimha – The half-lion, half-man avatar of Vishnu, fierce protector
Tava – Your
Da – Give (command form)
So Hum – I am That (a powerful yogic affirmation of unity with the Divine)

Narasimha, grant me your strength.
I am That (Divine).

This mantra invokes Narasimha, the half man, lion-headed incarnation of Vishnu in his inconquerable aspect, which provides protection, destruction of evil, and inner strength. This mantra brings powerful aegis as it identifies with Divine protection, invoking the Narasimha energy from within as a conscious force to destroy fear and inner demons, and activate fortitude.

I call this the "bad neighbor" mantra because it's especially effective when your energetic field is being disturbed – whether by loud neighbors, negative people, toxic energy, black magic, or disruptive influences. Chanting "Narasimha Ta Va Da So Hum" helps clear these disturbances swiftly. It's simple to repeat and powerful in moments of fear, psychic attack, emotional vulnerability, or any time you feel unsafe or energetically unsettled.

This mantra ignites courage, resolve, and divine fire to face both inner and outer challenges. It is a potent tool for karmic clearing, helping to dissolve deep-rooted patterns, ancestral imprints, and subconscious or past-life traumas. Through the "So Hum" vibration, it anchors the presence of the Higher Self, awakening spiritual empowerment, fierce devotion, and alignment with Divine Truth.

Chanting "Narasimha Ta Va Da So Hum" offers powerful proactive protection and is especially beneficial before engaging in spiritual practices, psychic readings, or mediumistic work, as it shields against astral interference. One of its most potent applications is in preventing nightmares, as Narasimha is not only a fierce protector but also a guardian of the subtle realms, defending the psyche from dark forces, fear projections, and subconscious intrusions. This mantra acts as a spiritual shield, dissolving energy cords, attachments, black magic, curses, and other invasive entities. As the Divine Dissolver of Demons, Narasimha is invoked to clear psychic residue, guard sleep, and fortify the aura against negative astral influences.

I have recommended the mantra "Narasimha Ta Va Da So Hum" countless times because of its extraordinary power to protect, clear fear-based energies, and dissolve nightmares. One especially profound case involved my client's four-year-old son, Jeremy, who was experiencing intense, recurring night terrors. Each night, he would awaken screaming, reliving a vivid dream of dying in a fiery explosion inside a tall building. The trauma was relentless, and his family was desperate for relief.

During a reading with Jeremy's mother, I entered a trance state and received a clear vision: Jeremy had been a victim of the 9/11 attacks in his previous lifetime. His soul had reincarnated just two decades later, still carrying the raw imprint of that traumatic death, which was now surfacing in his sleep as unresolved soul memory.

I advised his mother to chant "Narasimha Ta Va Da So Hum" each night after putting him to bed. This mantra, which calls on the fierce protective power of Lord Narasimha, acts as a shield for the psyche, especially during vulnerable states like sleep.

Remarkably, within four nights of his mother's consistent chanting, Jeremy's night terrors ceased entirely. The entire household finally began to rest peacefully. Six months later, his nightmares had not returned.

This case remains a powerful testament to the healing reach of sacred sound formulas of Sanskrit mantras, and how when used with intention and devotion – can cross the boundaries of time, lifetimes, and even death, to restore peace.

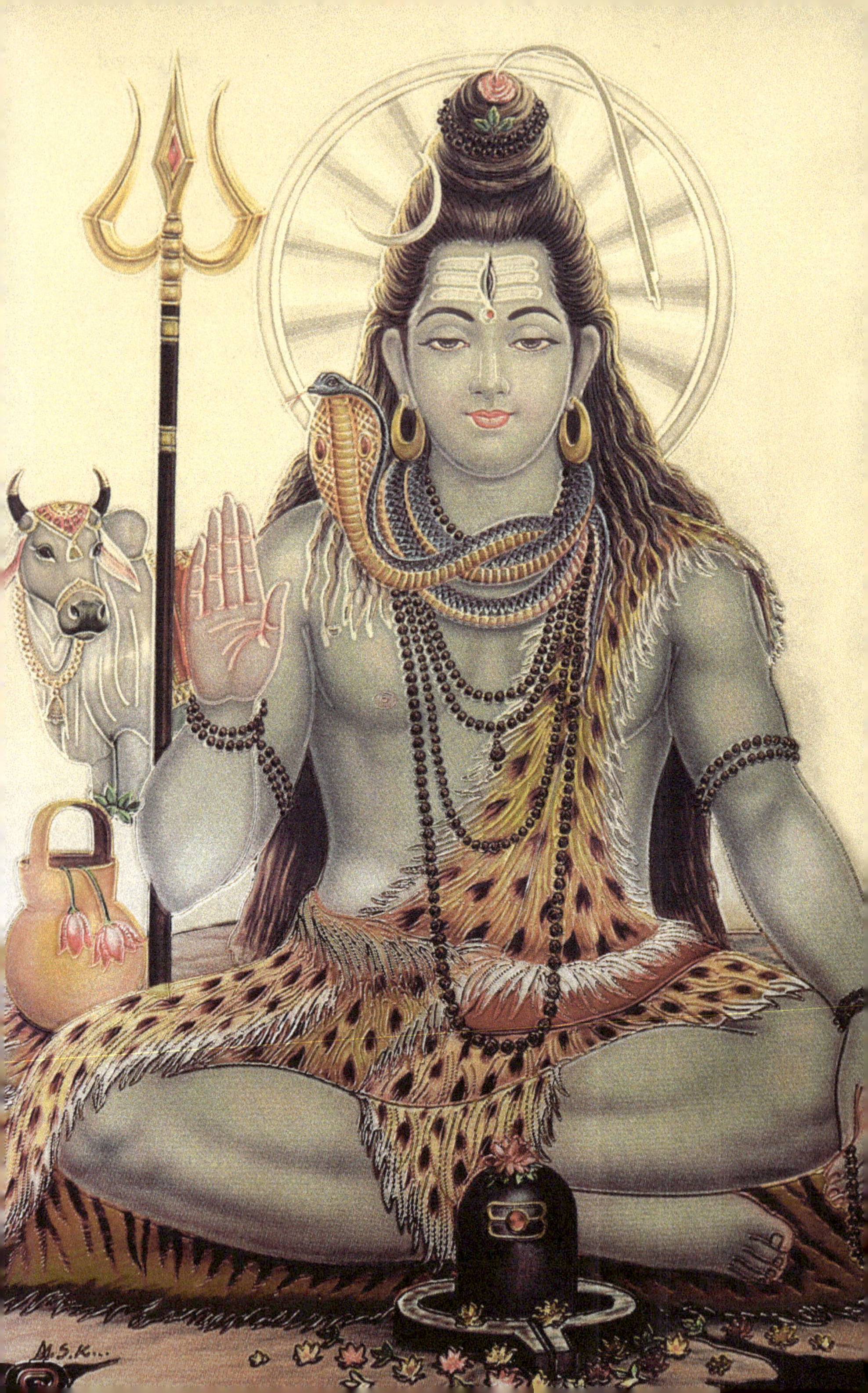
M.S.K...

9
Mantras for Liberation

The Shiva and Vishnu Principles

Now we come to mantras for liberation, or *moksha* – the ultimate aim of life according to Vedic philosophy. While *moksha* is traditionally associated with the final stage of the soul's journey, one does not have to wait until old age or renunciation to begin this practice. In fact, the earlier one begins chanting *moksha* mantras, the deeper the soul connection that can be cultivated over a lifetime.

Unlike mantras for *artha* (material prosperity) or *kama* (desire), *moksha* mantras are not about gaining anything external. They are about releasing illusion, shedding false identity, and reclaiming your true essence. These mantras are not based on belief – they are based on resonance. When you chant, you are not asking for liberation; you are activating it.

Chanting *moksha* mantras is like tuning a radio to the frequency of your soul. At first, the signal may seem faint or distant, but with consistent practice, it becomes clearer, stronger, and eventually unmistakable – until you remember that you are, and have always been, free, eternal and divine. Chanting Sanskrit liberation or *moksha* mantras is a profound spiritual practice rooted in thousands of years of yogic and Vedic tradition. These mantras – such as "Om

Namah Shivaya," "Om Namo Narayanaya," or "Om Mani Padme Hum" – are not just Sanskrit mantras that have stood the test of time, but vibrational codes that affect the body, mind, and soul on subtle and transformative levels. These mantras carry the frequency of liberation, gently dissolving the inner weight of burden and bringing clarity to the mind. Liberation mantras work on the causal plane of consciousness – the subtle layer where karmas, *samskaras* (soul impressions), and subconscious patterns reside. Through consistent chanting, these deeply rooted imprints begin to dissolve, releasing the soul from the cycles of fear, attachment, and rebirth.

The mind thrives on repetition, and mantra provides a sacred focal point. Unlike random thoughts or worries, mantras entrain the mind into stillness. Many *moksha* mantras also invoke Divine Love or surrender, gently awakening *bhakti* (devotion) and compassion. One may feel expanded love, forgiveness, or a release from the grip of the thinking mind.

With consistent chanting of liberation mantras, a profound sense of inner peace gradually unfolds, accompanied by increased emotional resilience and a subtle yet unmistakable freedom from old triggers. Karmic knots begin to unravel one by one, allowing the soul to awaken to its inherent, boundless freedom. These *moksha* mantras gently quiet the mind and open the heart, guiding the practitioner toward true liberation.

Additional benefits of chanting liberation mantras include the gradual shedding of layers of false identity, allowing the authentic Self to emerge. Reactivity softens, giving way to a deepening sense of peace and expanded awareness. Spiritual growth unfolds with increasing momentum, often marked by a rise in meaningful synchronicities. A subtle yet potent vibrational shield develops, providing resilience against external negativity and life's inevitable challenges.

Shiva

As Shiva represents the pure consciousness of God, Shiva mantras are commonly chanted to evolve one's individual consciousness and ultimately re-merge with the consciousness of Source. In the Vedic tradition, individual existence is seen as a cosmic game of peekaboo, in that Consciousness is hiding from itself and then revealing itself through the fractal perspective of separation. Existence can be likened to a dream. The dreamer experiences their dream from an individual perspective and encounters environments and other beings that seem to be separate from them. Yet the dream is ultimately a creation of the dreamer, so the beings and worlds that one encounters in one's dream are actually just manifestations of one's own consciousness seen through the illusion of separation.

The ultimate point of existence from the Vedic perspective is for Consciousness to better know itself.

Pure Consciousness or Shiva creates the cosmic dream of the universe then divides itself into all different conscious beings and enters the dream, willingly choosing to forget that it is the dreamer. The game now is to remember, to fully experience the process of evolving from one's illusory identity as a separate being to a spark of the fire of Universal Consciousness, a drop in the ocean of Being. Shiva mantras speed the process of remembering one's True Self, reconnecting with Source, and become a fully self-actualized individual manifestation of Divinity expressing itself on Earth through a human body and mind.

The idea of transcendental unity between the individual and Divine Consciousness is expressed across various spiritual traditions. For example, a mystical interpretation of when Jesus Christ said "I and The Father are one" is that Christ embodied this fully self-actualized state of being merged with Divine Consciousness. Essentially Christ woke up from the cosmic dream without dying; he realized he was dreaming while still remaining within the dream. His mission was to teach humanity how to do the same. Those of us who seek to follow "the way, the truth, and the light" of Christ would do well to follow his example by evolving our individual consciousness through acts of good karma (treat others as you'd like to be treated) and surrender of the limited ego identity and its desires to the will of God through prayer and meditation. Followers of the Vedic tradition see no contradiction between the teachings of Christ and the teachings of the Vedic seers – after all, truth is one, though many are its names. Sanskrit mantra as a concentrated form of energy-based prayer practice can help us to actualize the teachings of Christ, Buddha, and other mystical beings. Shiva mantras, including "Om Namah Shivaya," are simple yet powerful ways to evolve back into our original state of pure Being, Consciousness, and Bliss.

vishnu

Vishnu, one of the principal deities of the Vedic pantheon, is widely revered as the Preserver and Protector of the universe. While his primary role is to maintain cosmic order (*dharma*), Vishnu is also deeply associated with liberation (*moksha*) – the ultimate freedom from the cycle of birth, death, and rebirth (**samsara**).

Through his incarnations (avatars), Vishnu descends to Earth to restore balance whenever *adharma* (chaos and injustice) threatens the natural order. These avatars – such as Rama and Krishna – embody divine qualities that guide devotees toward righteousness, spiritual awakening, and liberation. Vishnu's grace is considered the bridge between human struggle and divine liberation, offering mercy and protection on the soul's journey home.

In the Vedic pantheon, Vishnu is part of the Trimurti, alongside Brahma the Creator and Shiva the Destroyer. While Brahma initiates creation and Shiva oversees transformation and dissolution, Vishnu maintains continuity and harmony. His role as Preserver connects all aspects of existence, making him central to sustaining life and spiritual balance.

Vishnu's connection with liberation is related to his compassionate nature. He guides souls toward *moksha* not through destruction or creation alone but through steady preservation of *dharma* and grace-filled intervention when necessary.

Within the Vedic tradition, Vishnu's power is inseparable from the Divine Feminine, often personified by his consort Lakshmi, the goddess of wealth, prosperity, and spiritual abundance. Lakshmi is not only the source of material fortune but also the embodiment of divine grace, which facilitates spiritual progress and liberation.

Lakshmi's presence beside Vishnu symbolizes the essential balance of masculine and feminine energies – the dynamic interplay of preservation and nurturing, power and compassion – that sustains the cosmos and supports the soul's evolution. Through this union, Vishnu's preservation extends beyond worldly order to include the nurturing of the soul's ultimate freedom.

om bhakta ganapatayei namaha

Om Bhak-tah Gah-nah-pah-tah-yei Nahm-ah-ha

Om – Sacred sound
Bhakta – Devotee, devotional
Ganapatayei – To Lord Ganesha
Namaha – I bow

Salutations to Ganesha, who is devoted to his devotees and removes their obstacles.

This mantra invokes Ganesha in his devotional form to remove obstacles for one on a spiritual path. In *Lord Ganesha*, Sadguru Sant Keshavadas recommends, "those who want enlightenment and *moksha* (liberation) should meditate on the pure white colored Ganesha while chanting the mantra, 'Om Bhakta Ganapatayei Namaha.'"*

This mantra will remove obstacles before starting a spiritual sadhana or devotional practice. Chanting it can help develop a deeper connection to the Divine. It will remove obstacles like procrastination or fear or doubt that interfere with performing spiritual practices such as meditation or chanting. It can strengthen the feeling of being guided and protected on your journey.

* Sadguru Sant Keshavadas, *Lord Ganesha* (Vishwa Dharma Publications, 1988), 28.

I share "Om Bhakta Ganapatayei Namaha," before a meditation at the end of the yoga classes that I teach. The group will chant it 9 or 27 times, leading into a silent meditation. Students have given me feedback that they go into very deep meditations. Some have felt energy and vibration moving in different chakras after chanting this mantra. One student told me she felt a popping sensation in her third eye, saw an explosion of purple, and started seeing images like she was watching a movie of herself. Another student reported warmth in her heart, and then light blue energy in her third eye and then saw a blue Shiva appear. Several students have seen Ganesha appear, some in yellow, orange or gold, and felt his *darshan* and blessings.

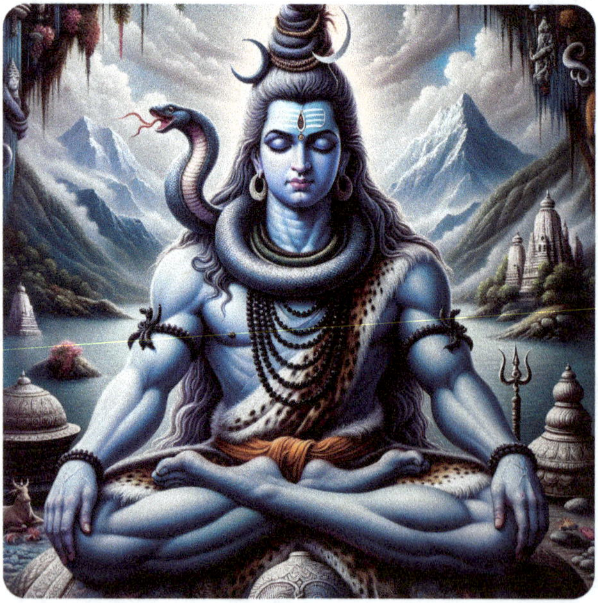

om namah shivaya

Om Nah-mah Shee-vah-yah

Om – Sacred sound
Namaha – I bow
Shivaya – To Shiva

I bow to Lord Shiva, the auspicious, benevolent one – the inner Self and pure consciousness.

"Om Namah Shivaya" is one of the oldest known Sanskrit mantras, tracing its written origins to the Yajurveda, one of the four Vedas (foundational texts of the Vedic tradition). "Om Namah Shivaya" is also the foundational mantra of the Shaivite tradition, marked by those who view Shiva as their preferred form of God. Shiva represents pure Consciousness, the sum total and wellspring of all individual forms of consciousness in the universe, from primitive bacteria to divine beings. Shiva, or Consciousness, interacts with its counterpart Shakti (Matter and Energy) to create the universe. The Consciousness of Shiva is depicted as the masculine polarity of existence while Shakti represents the feminine polarity. Together, these archetypal energies create, maintain, and destroy all aspects of creation through their cosmic dance.

Shiva mantras are very effective for hastening our spiritual evolution. "Om Namah Shivaya" in particular does this by aligning us with the pure Consciousness of God represented as Shiva and named in the mantra. However, the mantras syllables also work directly with the five archetypal elements of creation: Earth (Na), Water (Ma), Fire (Shi), Air (Va), Ether (Ya). These five syllables represent the five symbolic elements that make up the universe and the human body. The elements also correspond with the first five core chakras along the spine, as each chakra is considered to be ruled by one of these five elements. The additional starting syllable of "Om" corresponds with the archetypal element of Mind and is associated with the sixth chakra, the Third Eye. When all of these six archetypal elements of creation and their associated chakras are in harmonious energetic alignment within an individual, merging with the Consciousness of Divinity happens naturally. Chanting "Om Namah Shivaya" purifies these elements within ourselves and connects us directly to the divine energy of Source. The individual retains their individual self, yet willingly forgoes attachment to that limited identity, having reached the state of Enlightenment, sometimes referred to as Christ Consciousness. Such a person is a blessing to themselves and to all of humanity.

As a yoga teacher and mantra instructor, I have led many groups in chanting the **Siddha** mantra, "Om Namah Shivaya." During these sessions, students have shared remarkable experiences – some feeling the powerful presence of Shiva in the room, as if receiving his *darshan* (blessing) directly. Others have described visions of deep indigo or brilliant shades of blue, the sacred colors associated with Shiva energy.

One of my students entered a deep meditation while chanting this mantra, and had a compelling vision of Shiva in his Rudra form, stirring a blue cauldron. In that moment, she received an inner message that everything would work out. At the time she had been under great stress from a legal situation directed against her. Remarkably just days after this profound Shiva chant and meditation, the issue was resolved and she was left free and clear.

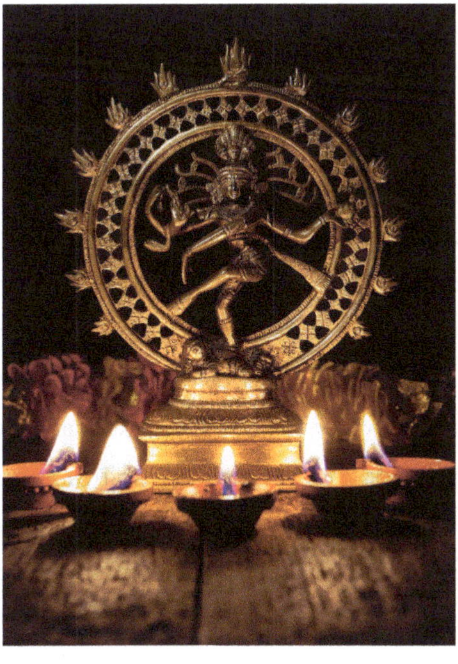

om namo bhagavate vasudevaya

Om Nah-mo Bhah-gah-vah-teh Vah-soo-day-vah-yah

Om – Sacred sound
Namo – Salutations
Bhagavate – To the Lord
Vasudevaya – To Vasudeva (Krishna, the son of Vasudeva)

Salutations to the Lord Vasudeva, the indwelling divine presence (Krishna).

This mantra is also interpreted as "Om and Salutations to the indwelling one. Oh infinite Lord, indweller in the heart of all beings, unto you do I turn my consciousness." It leads us to see God within everyone and everything. It is a powerful invocation of Vishnu through Lord Krishna, to cultivate devotion (*bhakti*), surrender, and spiritual awakening.

As a mantra of liberation, it offers profound spiritual guidance toward attaining *moksha* or *mukti* – the ultimate freedom from samsara, the endless cycle of birth and death. This 12-syllable mantra is revered as one of the foremost Vishnu mantras, often called the supreme mantra and celebrated as the hymn of liberation. It is traditionally recited as a powerful tool for achieving spiritual emancipation and release from worldly bondage. As its sacred sound reverberates, it dissolves the illusions binding the spirit, guiding the seeker into the timeless realm of infinite peace and radiant transcendence. Because of its profound power to inspire equanimity and elevation, this mantra is often chanted during meditation, prayer, or devotional singing (*kirtan*). It soothes the mind, purifies the heart, and gently opens the path to self-realization. It is revered as a mantra of protection, guidance, and divine grace, supporting the seeker in transcending ego, dissolving illusion, and easing suffering through wholehearted surrender to the supreme will.

Interestingly, this mantra not only has the power to liberate the soul during embodiment but can also support the incarnation of an enlightened soul for a woman who wishes to conceive or is already pregnant.

This sacred mantra has guided many into deeper states of meditation and communion with the Divine. For over two decades, I've offered it to women in the early stages of pregnancy as a way to call in an enlightened soul. Time and again, they've been blessed with children who carry a rare light – beings of wisdom, sensitivity, and spiritual depth.

om namo narayanaya

Om Nah-mo Nah-rah-yah-nah-yah

Om – Sacred sound
Namo – Salutations
Narayana – The all-pervading divine (Vishnu)
Ya – To

Salutations to Narayana, the supreme protector and sustainer of the universe.

"Salutations to the Divine Presence that dwells in all beings." "Om Namo Narayanaya" is a powerful Vishnu mantra and a mantra of peace, surrender, and divine alignment. It is known as a *shanti* mantra (mantra of peace) and is often used to invoke inner stillness, divine protection, and spiritual awakening. This sacred mantra calls upon the preserving power of Vishnu to guide the soul through life's thresholds – especially the great transition of death. It is said to open a luminous path for the soul, ensuring a serene, swift, and divinely held passage into the next realm.

This mantra serves as a formidable aid during times of transition, especially the final journey of death, offering ease, grace, and spiritual support throughout the process. If a loved one, including a cherished animal companion, is nearing the end of life, chanting this mantra can help ease their passage, offering peace, comfort, and a gentle transition. In Vedic tradition, by chanting this mantra one will reach the spiritual abode of Lord Vishnu or Narayana. Vaikuntha is a realm beyond the material world, full of bliss (**ananda**), peace (*shanti*), and eternal existence (*sat*).

Narayana is seen as a protector of *dharma* and the soul's journey. The mantra invokes his grace for support through life's challenges. Chanting this mantra helps align the individual self with universal consciousness, fostering a deep sense of unity, inner peace, and divine trust. It quiets the mind, soothes emotional turbulence, and anchors the practitioner in a state of stillness and surrender. As the mantra dissolves ego-driven thoughts and emotions, it cultivates humility and attunement to the divine will. It can help one reach a state of liberated consciousness, where the soul abides in unity with the Divine, free from karma and rebirth. This can be an inner spiritual state where the mind is beyond duality and suffering – an awakened state of being. It doesn't necessarily mean that one has to die to attain it.

In yogic and Ayurvedic traditions, this mantra is also used for energetic healing, believed to harmonize the subtle body – particularly the heart and crown chakras. With steady repetition and devotion, it is said to purify karma, support spiritual awakening, and ultimately guide the soul toward liberation from the cycle of rebirth.

I have chanted this mantra many times as people are in the process of passing away. When our beloved teacher, Namadeva, was leaving his body on October 1, 2010, many of his devotees around the world were chanting "Om Namo

Narayanaya" for his smooth journey to the higher realms, known as Vaikuntha. I told him to give me a message when he arrived. That evening the light by my bedside turned on randomly in the middle of the night. I turned it off, and it turned on again. I realized that was Namadeva's signal to me that he had made it to the final destination.

My most profound experience of chanting "Om Namo Narayanaya" was when my husband was dying at Massachusetts General Hospital. The doctors had done all they could, but his organs were shutting down, and it was clear he was in the final stages of leaving his body. Once he was removed from life support, I instinctively began chanting "Om Namo Narayanaya" and "Om Mani Padme Hum."

Though he could no longer speak, he could hear me – and a gentle smile spread across his face. I sat at his bedside, holding his hand, chanting these sacred mantras without pause for nearly five hours, holding vigil as he transitioned. There was only one nurse present during that time, and she quietly said, "I don't know what you're saying or doing, but it feels incredibly peaceful in here."

As I continued chanting, I suddenly felt a surge of energy move from his hand into mine – like a wave of warmth and love flooding through me. He also transmitted warmth and pulses of energy directly into my heart. My heart chakra began to buzz and expand, as if it were being lit from within. I turned to the nurse and described what I was experiencing.

She nodded and said softly, "He's filling you with his love – and the last of his life force."

Then his heart stopped beating – he flatlined – though surprisingly, he was still breathing. I turned to the nurse and asked why he was still breathing if his heart had stopped. She replied gently, "It happens sometimes, but the official time of death is marked when the heart stops."

As I sat with that, a deeper understanding washed over me. Years ago, we had first met when I was his breathwork teacher. It struck me – he was showing me, in his own final gesture of devotion and humor, that even in death, he was still breathing like the dedicated breathwork student he had once been.

The moment I had that realization... his breath, too, ceased.

I knew with certainty that the mantras had helped guide his soul to a higher spiritual realm. The vibrations created a tunnel of love and light for his departure. A few days later, he appeared to me in a dream, beaming with gratitude. He thanked me for helping him leave his body, saying the mantras had carried him through that long tunnel of light with my voice and love.

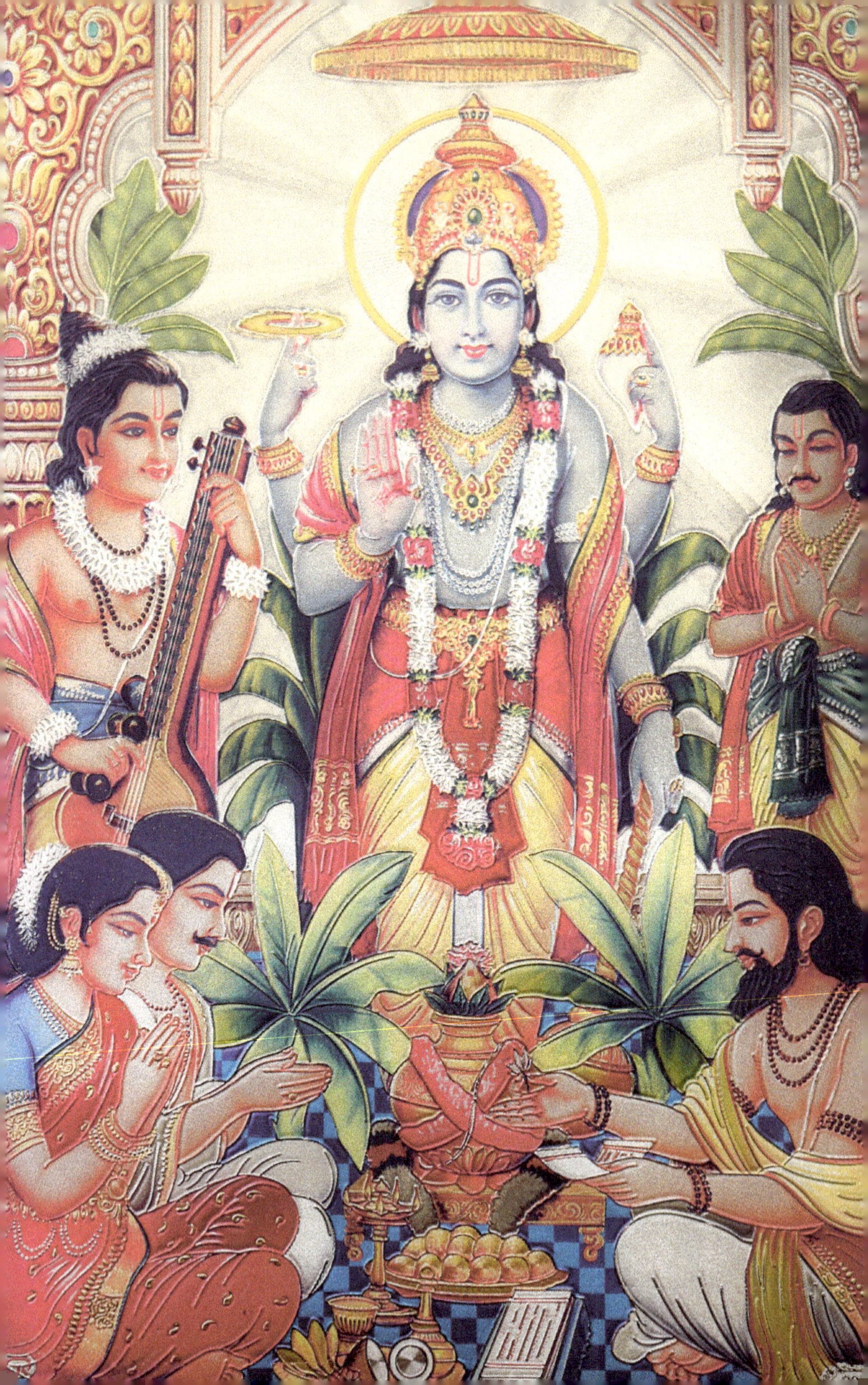

Om Mani Padme Hum

Om Ma-nee Pad-may Hoom

Om – Sacred sound
Mani – Jewel
Padme – Lotus
Hum – Seal of the heart, unity, and protection

The jewel is in the lotus.

The lotus "padme" symbolizes purity, spiritual unfolding, and enlightenment, growing from the mud yet untainted.The jewel represents compassion, wisdom, and an awakened heart.

In Tibetan Buddhism, this sacred mantra is often inscribed on stones, etched into prayer wheels, and printed on fluttering prayer flags throughout the Himalayan regions. It is believed that simply seeing, hearing, or reciting "Om Mani Padme Hum" bestows blessings and invokes the compassionate presence of Avalokiteshvara.

Each of the six syllables corresponds to one of the six realms of existence in Buddhist cosmology. As the mantra is chanted, it is said to purify the karmic causes that bind beings to these realms, supporting liberation from the cycle of rebirth.

Chanting this mantra gently invokes compassion – for yourself and for others. It is especially soothing during times of emotional pain, fear, or grief, offering a sense of comfort and connection. When incorporated into meditation, "Om Mani Padme Hum" helps open the heart and dissolve layers of judgment, softening the mind and spirit.

Because of its profound spiritual vibration, this mantra generates a powerful field of loving presence – not only for the one chanting, but for anyone nearby. It can be especially supportive for those who are dying or suffering, as I shared in the testimonial involving "Om Namo Narayanaya." Reciting "Om Mani Padme Hum" also supports the purification of karmic imprints, helping to bring deep peace to both the mind and the surrounding environment.

Om Mani Padme Hum

by Dr. Alexi Jardine Martel

"Om Mani Padme Hum" is the most widely chanted mantra in the world. It comes from the Buddhist tradition and invokes the energy of Avalokiteshvara, the Buddha of Compassion. Sometimes it is pronounced differently among certain Buddhist traditions, but here it is given in the original Sanskrit. The sound transliteration of the mantra is "Om Manee Pad-may Hoom." The syllables of the mantra break down to "Om" (the cosmic sound of oneness – creation, preservation, and destruction in one)

"Mani" (which refers to the conscious mind, or more specifically the decision-making and thinking faculties of the individual) "Padme" (which refers to the heart, or the emotional and feeling core of the individual) and "Hum" (a seed sound which enhances and projects the energy of the throat chakra, the seat of will and authority of speech). Together the mantra works to link the mind with the heart in a powerful way, connecting them through the conduit of manifestation through speech that is the throat. In this way, the mantra activates and illuminates the higher chakras of the individual – heart, throat, and head – thereby powerfully uplifting one's consciousness to higher states of being.

Compassion is a term we hear a lot these days and it appears in many spiritual traditions, sometimes given as synonymous with Love. "Om Mani Padme Hum" is the mantra of compassion. It serves to increase compassion in the individual. However, like all mantras, any description of its effects or a breakdown of the meaning of its syllables fails to encapsulate the true meaning of a mantra. Like fire or wind, a mantra must be experienced in life for it to be truly understood.

From my experiences chanting this mantra through a 40-day discipline, I can attest to its power. Honestly, this mantra surprised me. I began chanting it with a desire to enhance compassion within myself, which I vaguely believed to mean the mantra would make me nicer. After all, we all could be a little nicer these days. However, what I experienced when working deeply with this mantra was a profound sense of inner peace, as my often restless mind was soothed by the increasingly sublime connection with the heart. The mantra enhanced the sense of being held by the Divine, that everything is and would be okay. It created a sanctuary of stillness like the calm of the deep ocean undisturbed by the sometimes stormy surface. In a practical sense, the mantra did help to make me nicer. I found the energy of the mantra to be the opposite of anger, as it invoked a tranquility that quelled agitation. When dealing with the day-to-day frustrations of traffic, the occasional unpleasantness of strangers, or the pressures of work and money, this mantra served as a beacon of peace.

I also found that the Mani mantra improved my feelings toward strangers and humanity in general. It's not uncommon these days to look upon the world and find humanity to be lacking. Through the perceived immoral behaviors of individuals to the rampant greed and destruction at the societal level, there is a lot for one to get upset over. This is likely not an accident, as forces that oppose the spiritual evolution of humanity seek to divide and conquer us by playing to the lesser angels of the ego such fear, anger, and greed. Such forces seek to not only spread such divisive energies but also enhance the perception that such darkness is more prevalent than it actually is. Compare an hour of watching the nightly news and the feelings it stirs in you about the world and your fellow humans to the feelings of walking an hour in a public park. The goodness of the world is freely available to us if we have the courage to bravely venture into our surroundings with an open mind and open heart. The weavers of illusion seek to close our minds and hearts and keep us trapped in our own isolated worlds through the narratives they spread. Sanskrit mantras are an energetic force of the Divine that elevate us and quicken our spiritual evolution. Against such instruments of divinity, darkness cannot hold. Mantras in general provide a form of spiritual armor, called *Kavacha*, that protects the individual from forces that would seek to delude or control them. Mantras even protect us from our own inner darkness, which the outer darkness seeks to hook into in order to control us. The mantra "Om Mani Padme Hum" purifies our inner being as well as radiates powerful compassion into the world, thus neutralizing both inner and outer darkness. This mantra is a powerful tool for connecting with the True Source and bringing about spiritual transformation at both a personal and collective level. Saying it helps to calm the mind and transcend fear, anger, anxiety, and other negative energetic states. It grants spiritual growth with greater happiness and inner peace for both you and the world. Chant the Sanskrit mantra "Om Mani Padme Hum" and better embody your own aspect of Divinity here on Earth.

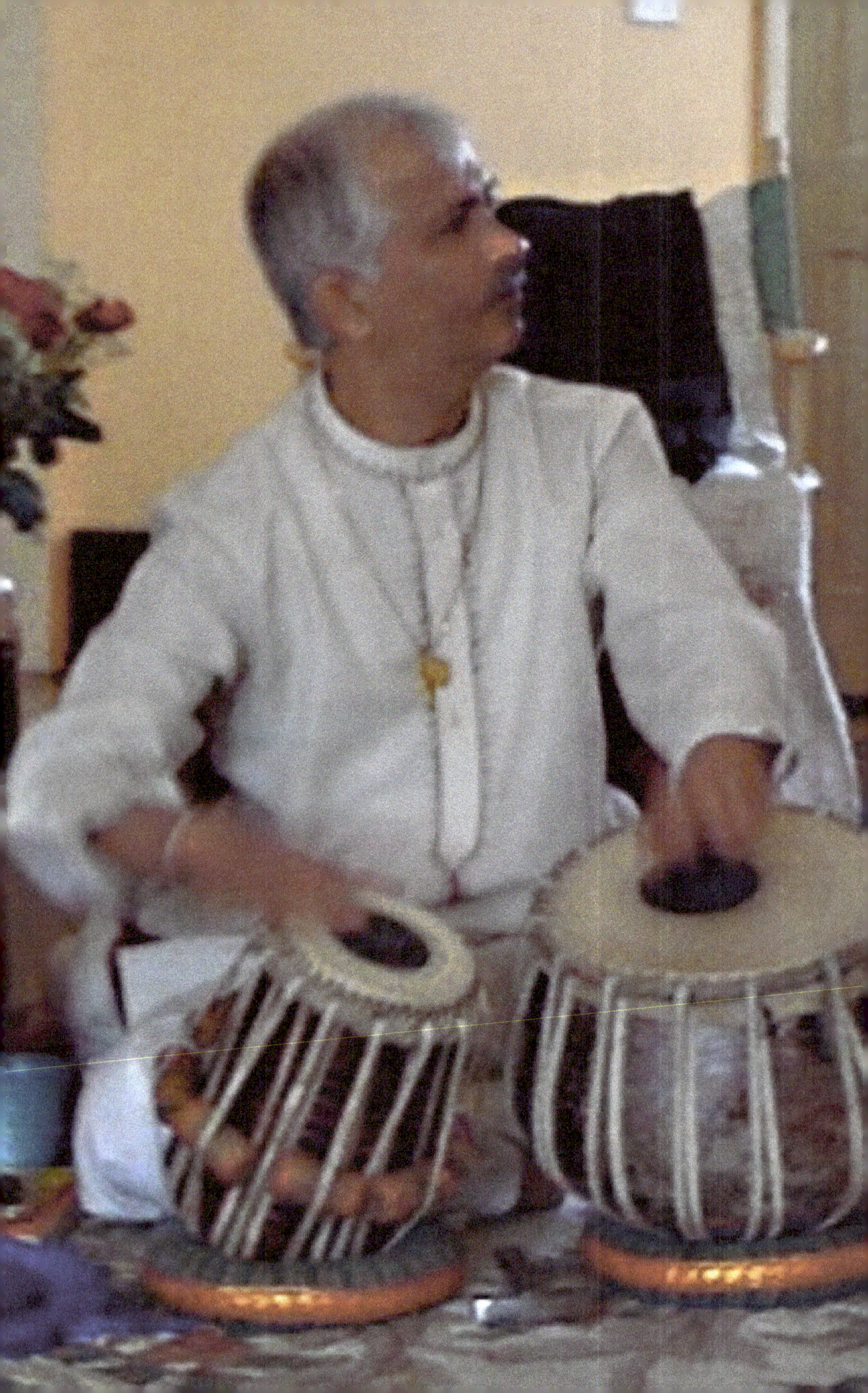

10
Muraliji's Story

Sri Muralidhar Pai, son of mantra gurus Sadguru Sant Keshavadas and Guru Rama Mata, was raised in their spiritual tradition alongside his sister Geeta and brother Shyam. Growing up in a household unlike any other, they experienced a profoundly unconventional life.

Sant Keshavadas, founder of the Temple of Cosmic Religion, descended from an ancient lineage of singing saints and embodied the path of **Bhakti Yoga**, or devotional mysticism. He established numerous temples and meditation centers across the United States, including the Bhagavad-Gita Mandir and Gayatri University in Bangalore, India. Throughout his life, he led over thirty peace pilgrimages worldwide, dedicating himself wholeheartedly to the cause of world peace. As the author of more than 45 books and composer of over 45,000 spiritual songs in Sanskrit and other languages, his profound legacy continues through the unwavering devotion of his wife and the divine spark of God-realization he awakened in his disciples and followers. His books can be found in the bibliography.

Muraliji shares his journey in the following narrative.

My father and mother were my first and foremost gurus. His lifestyle was unlike any other household because he was always deeply attuned to Panduranga – a name meaning "bright light," which refers to the divine self. Panduranga is also called Vitthala, symbolizing the entire Trinity. The word breaks down as follows: "Vi" represents the Creator, "Tha" refers removing all poison and negativity from the world, embodying Ishwara (Shiva), "La" signifies Lakshmi, and "Khanta" refers to Lakshmi's consort, Vishnu. This sacred name carries profound significance.

My father continuously chanted the divine name of Vitthala. From childhood, my siblings and I were raised differently than most children. Our home was always filled with meditation, chanting of stotras, recitations of the Vedas and Upanishads, and the writing of spiritual books. This upbringing made me realize early on that our lifestyle was far from ordinary – it was a unique form of guruhood, completely distinct from any other.

As I grew, I listened to stories from the Ramayana, the Mahabharata, the Bhagavad Gita, and teachings from saints across India – all of which my father carried within him and shared with us. It wasn't just about whispering mantras in our ears as babies; the sacred sounds and mantras were a living presence in our daily lives.

My father would chant mantras like "Om Namo Bhagavate Vasudevaya" and "Om Namo Bhagavate Panduranga," nurturing us spiritually as we grew. My brother and I are seven years apart, while my sister is about one and a half years younger than me. Our names were chosen with deep meaning: our father's name was Keshava, a name of Lord Krishna, meaning "the one with curly locks of hair."

Before marriage, my mother was named Nirmala, but my father renamed her Rama, symbolizing Lakshmi or Rukmini, Krishna's consort. As for me, I was named Murali Dhar, which means "the holder of the flute" – a direct reference to Krishna, who plays the flute to enchant and guide. "Murali" means flute, and "Dhar" means bearer or holder.

This naming was no coincidence – it was a reflection of the deep spiritual lineage and devotion that shaped our family and my own path.

From a young age, I traveled and performed alongside my father before large audiences – crowds unlike any I had ever seen. One of the most memorable moments was playing at the Rashtrapati Bhavan, the official residence of the President of India. At that time, Dr. Sarvepalli Radhakrishnan was serving as President, and he had personally invited my father to Delhi for a special performance.

Back in Bangalore, my father had also inaugurated the beautiful Panduranga Mandir in Rajajinagar, a significant spiritual center. The event was graced by the presence of the Maharaja of Mysore, who officially opened our ashram, lending his royal support. It was a moment of great honor and recognition for our work and devotion.

Having the blessings of such revered figures as President Radhakrishnan and the Maharaja affirmed the deep spiritual and cultural significance of our path, and I was privileged to witness and be part of these profound experiences from an early age.

My father authored 45 books in multiple languages, encompassing the wisdom of saints from all over India. He was deeply immersed in the devotional traditions of both the South and North, chanting bhajans composed by revered saints such as the Purandara Dasa lineage from the South and iconic figures like Tukaram, Meera Bai, Sant Dnyaneshwar, and Sant Namdev from the North. He also honored the lady saints – Mirabai and others – who devoted their lives entirely to Krishna, the one without a second.

His devotion centered on Panduranga, regarded as Krishna himself before his departure to the Supreme. Panduranga embodies the final awakening of Kundalini energy before the onset of the Kali Yuga.

My father carried within him the vast reservoir of knowledge from the Vedas, Upanishads, Bhagavad Gita, Ramayana, and countless other spiritual texts. This wisdom was not acquired through conventional study; it was an intrinsic part of his being. Similarly, I never formally studied tabla or harmonium – these gifts manifested naturally within me, just as my father played the harmonium flawlessly without a formal teacher. His teacher was Saraswati, the goddess of wisdom and learning, from whom he received direct inspiration. My father received his knowledge directly from Saraswati, the goddess of wisdom and learning. Vidya, which means true knowledge, came to him naturally and effortlessly from a very young age – by the time he was just eight years old. To have such a father was nothing short of a divine blessing – a truly godly presence in my life.

I first met Namadeva when I was serving as a temple priest in Washington, D.C. My father brought him to the temple, and from the very beginning, Namadeva and I developed a close bond.

I began teaching him the proper rituals and ceremonies – starting with the Panduranga Puja. Together, we also performed Devi Puja, Janmashtami Puja, Krishna Puja, Rama Puja, and most notably, the Satyanarayana Puja. I guided Namadeva in conducting these pujas with the utmost reverence and precision.

Though we were colleagues as temple priests, our relationship grew into a deep friendship. Namadeva even honored me by serving as the best man at my wedding.

My father played a pivotal role in popularizing the Satyanarayana Puja in this country at a time when temples were scarce, bringing this sacred practice into the hearts of many.

From a young age, Muraliji traveled extensively with his father, performing *pujas* and absorbing the sacred mantras that formed the foundation of their spiritual path. Beginning at the age of 12, his journeys took him across Europe, the United States, Trinidad, and other countries – immersing him in diverse cultures while deepening his connection to his heritage.

His mother, Guru Rama Mata, learned alongside him and his father and excelled in Hari Katha, the divine storytelling tradition. After his father's passing in 1997, she led the Vishwa Shanti Ashram, continuing the family's spiritual mission despite great challenges.

Around 2010, Muraliji began traveling with his mother, carrying forward the legacy they had both nurtured. During this period, he met Parashakti Jill, who, at Namadeva's request, organized a spiritual gathering in the Boston area. The event featured Sanskrit mantras, *kirtan*, and sacred *puja* performed by the Gurus of the lineage. He attended alongside Guru Rama Mata, Namadeva, and Satyabhama. This gathering was more than a celebration – it symbolized the passing of the torch, a continuation of Namadeva's profound legacy, and a renewal of their shared spiritual journey.

The following pages share some of Muraliji's most cherished mantras – frequently recommended to his students for their potency and transformative effects.

om shri rama jaya rama jaya jaya rama

Om Shree Rah-mah Jai-yah
Rah-mah Jai-yah Jai-yah Rah-mah

Om – Sacred sound
Sri – Reverence, auspiciousness; Here, "Sri Rama" signifies the glorious, revered form of Lord Rama
Rama – The name of Lord Rama, the seventh incarnation of Vishnu. Represents truth, virtue, dharma, inner strength, and divine protection
Jaya – Means victory, glory, or triumph
Jaya Rama – Victory to Rama" or "Glory to Rama"

Om, O Auspicious Lord Rama, Victory to You, Victory to You Again and Again!

The repetition intensifies the energy: "Victory, victory to Rama!" and implies complete surrender, celebration, and affirmation of the divine power of Rama again and again. According to Muraliji's father, Sat Guru Sant Keshavadas, chanting the mantra "Om Sri Rama Jaya Rama Jaya Jaya Rama" bestows the same blessings as reciting the 1,008 names of Vishnu, known as the Vishnu Sahasranam. This makes it a profoundly potent mantra for clearing karma on multiple levels.

As Muraliji explains, the syllable "Ra" has the power to expel negative karma – as it is spoken, it is said to release harmful energies from the body, without disturbing the positive. The sound "Ma" acts as a seal, protecting the chanter from absorbing further negativity. Together, the vibrational force of Rama works to dissolve inner resistance and purify the subtle layers of the being.

This mantra is widely regarded as a *moksha*, or liberation mantra, as it supports the soul in crossing the ocean of death and rebirth, ultimately dissolving the grip of ego. A devotional powerhouse, it draws the awareness deep into the heart, anchoring the practitioner in presence and surrender. By invoking the name of Rama, it calls forth divine protection and aligns the individual with truth, righteousness, and the higher will. Through continued repetition, the chanter becomes attuned to the current of Divine Love, which leads the soul toward freedom.

When Muraliji has offered this mantra to his students, many have reported remarkable and even miraculous shifts in their lives. The name Rama, he explains, reveals the path of right living and noble character – it teaches us how to be truly human. Chanting this mantra not only uplifts the spirit but also acts as a shield, repelling negative influences and circumstances. Muraliji has witnessed individuals being almost mysteriously lifted out of difficult or toxic situations, guided by the protective grace of the mantra.

om sharavana bhavaya namaha

Om Shah-rah-vah-nah Bhah-vah-yah Nahm-ah-ha

Om – Sacred sound
Sharavana Bhava – Sharavana refers to the sacred reeds (Sharavana = "forest of reeds") from which Lord Murugan was born, according to legend. Bhava means being, essence, or state. Together, Sharavana Bhava refers to He who was born of the sacred Sharavana forest – the divine warrior and embodiment of purity, valor, wisdom, and spiritual victory.
Namaha – I bow

I bow to Lord Murugan, the embodiment of divine power and wisdom.

Lord Murugan, also known as Kartikeya, Skanda, or Subrahmanya, is the radiant son of Shiva and Parvati and the elder brother of Ganesha. Revered as the god of war, divine courage, and spiritual wisdom, he embodies the victory of light over darkness and higher consciousness over ignorance.

Namadeva frequently recommended this mantra, praising its ability to bring good fortune and auspicious outcomes. Muraliji describes it as a powerful remedy for life's sufferings, offering relief from mental distress, anxiety, and fear.

Chanting "Om Sharavana Bhavaya Namaha" invokes the protective grace of Lord Murugan and infuses the practitioner with clarity, courage, and inner strength. As the brother of Ganesha, Murugan also aids in removing obstacles – both material and spiritual. This mantra refines one's discernment, purifies the mind and senses, and dissolves negative karmic patterns, especially those rooted in ego, confusion, or delusion.

It also activates the third eye and throat chakras, enhancing intuition, insight, and authentic self-expression.

om sri sriyei namaha

Om Shree Shree-yei Nahm-ah-ha

Om – Sacred sound
Sri – Reverence, auspiciousness
Sriyei – To the goddess Sri Lakshmi
Namaha – I bow

Om, I bow to the auspicious, radiant divine feminine.

Chanting "Om Sri Sriyei Namaha" invokes the nurturing, graceful and prosperous aspects of Shakti (divine feminine power), especially in her Lakshmi form.

Muraliji teaches that this mantra brings material, spiritual, and mental wealth, bestowing both inner and outer abundance. Invoking Lakshmi as "Sri," the mantra draws in steady and consistent blessings, while also cultivating the mental resilience needed to pursue inspired ideas and manifest prosperity.

Lakshmi, as the goddess of both wealth and wisdom, guides individuals in creating abundance without losing spiritual grounding. Through her grace, wealth can arrive from multiple sources, while the mind remains strong and centered.

Chanting this mantra can also restore harmony in relationships and within the home, and supports the graceful unfolding of life events. In Shakti and Lakshmi-based traditions, it is often given to cultivate inner radiance, beauty, and magnetic presence, all aligned with one's *dharma* – the soul's right path.

om klim kalikayei namaha

Om Kleem Ka-lee-kai-yei Nahm-ah-ha

Om – Sacred sound
Klim – *Bija* mantra associated with attraction, transformation, and invocation of divine feminine energy. Klim is often linked with Krishna, Kali, and other deities, symbolizing magnetic power and spiritual potency.
Kalikayei – Kali is the fierce aspect of the Divine Mother (*Devi*), symbolizing destruction of ignorance, transformation, and liberation.
-yei suffix denotes "to Kali" or "for Kali," addressing or offering the mantra to the goddess Kali.
Namaha – I bow

Om, I bow to the divine Goddess Kali,
the fierce and transformative energy,
invoking her magnetic power and grace.

This mantra offers profound protection – both as a proactive shield and in moments of heightened vulnerability. It safeguards the chanter from negative energies, psychic interference, and harmful influences. More subtly, it dissolves egoic projections from others as well as the inner shadows within oneself. By invoking the Divine Mother in her fierce and transformative form as Kali, the mantra calls forth a force that cuts through ignorance, dissolves attachments, and clears the path for spiritual awakening.

The *bija* syllable "Klim" charges the mantra with magnetic power – drawing in divine grace and accelerating personal transformation. When chanted with devotion, the mantra awakens Kali's energy within: a force that liberates the soul by burning away fear, illusion, and limitation. It is a powerful ally for those walking the path of inner growth, courage, and freedom.

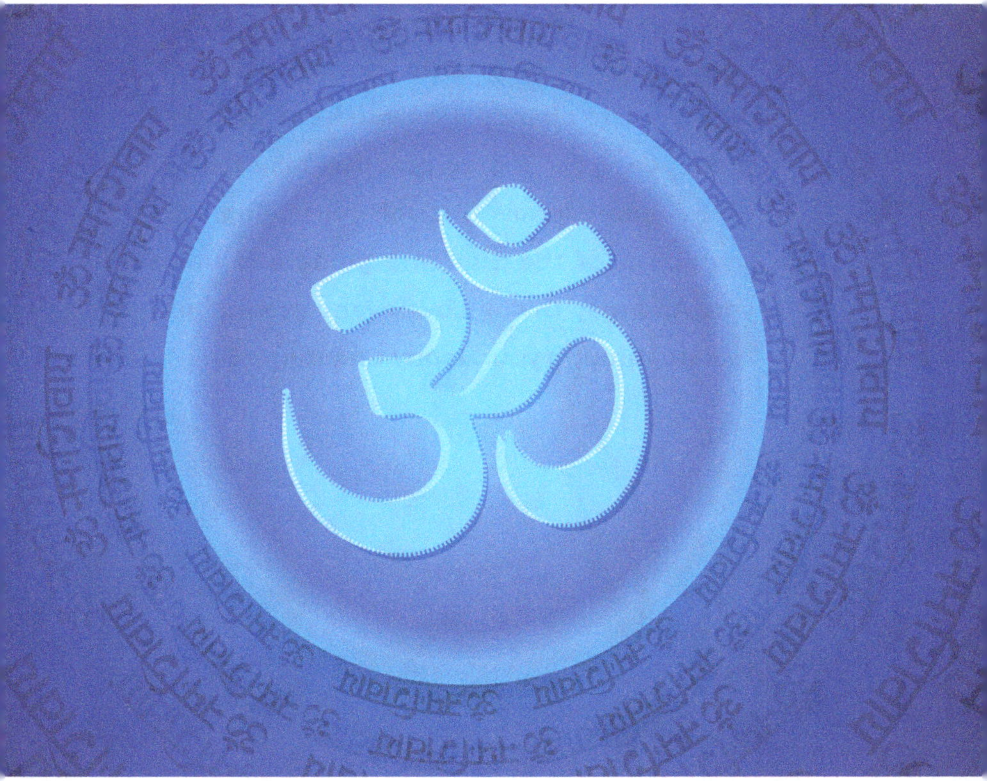

epilogue

May your efforts bear abundant fruit. It is our heartfelt wish that this book inspires you to begin your journey with Sanskrit mantra – or, if you are already a devoted chanter, that it deepens your sacred practice. May the joy of the universe flow through your being. May the power of the Supreme guide and uplift you. And may Divine Love ever surround and radiate through you. Happy Chanting!

"There is a saying in Sanskrit commonly said amongst spiritual teachers and priest in india,

'NAMA EVA, NAMA EVA, KEVALAM...'

The divine name alone,
the divine name alone,
brings freedom.

The divine name is a colloquial phrase
for a Sanskrit mantra."

~Namadeva Acharya

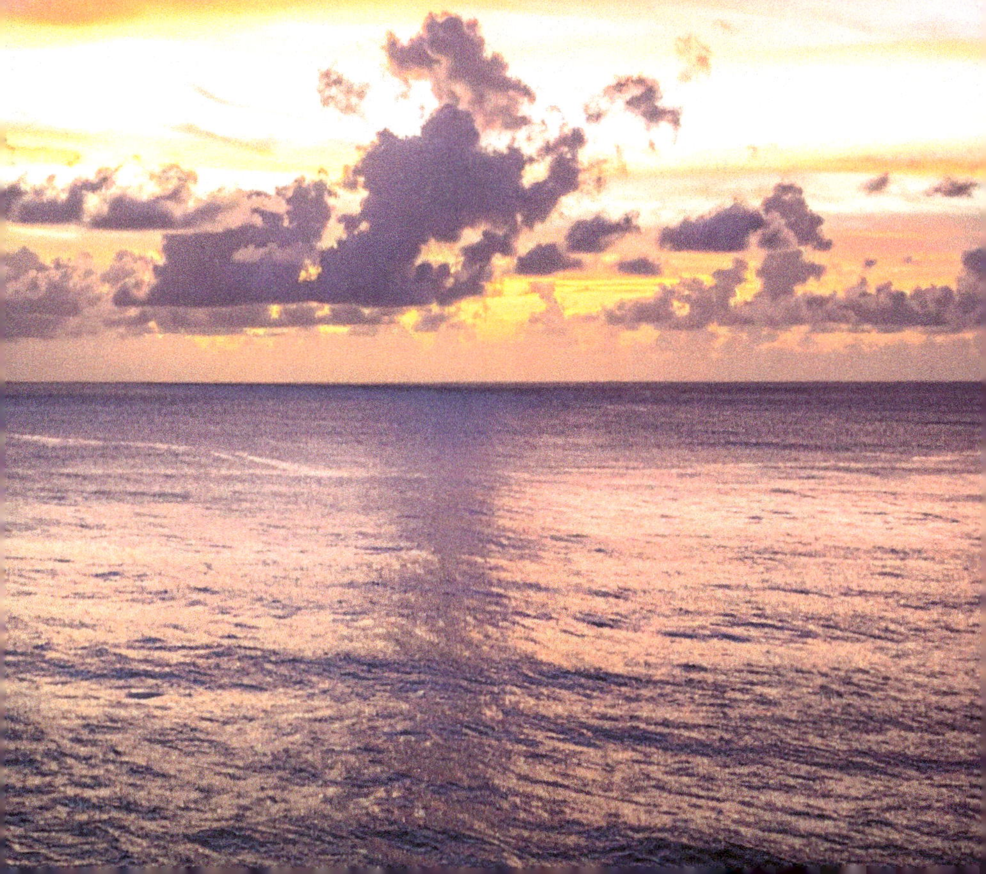

glossary & related terms

ADEPT Spiritually advanced being with esoteric abilities and knowledge.

ADVAITA Refers to a philosophy of non-dualism where everything, including all souls, is the same Being. This philosophy posits no difference between a soul and God.

AJAPA JAPA The effortless or unceasing repetition of a mantra.

AJNA CHAKRA Spiritual center between the eyebrows, often referred to as the sixth chakra or third eye, where the masculine and feminine currents of the body meet and join. The merging of the two currents produce an interior sound, "Om."

ANAHATA CHAKRA The spiritual heart center, also called the fourth chakra. It is where the descending triangle of the upper chakras (crown, third eye, and throat chakra descend to meet the lower three chakras of the root, naval, and solar plexus chakra).

ANANDA Bliss. Also, the final word in names of monks who have taken Sanyas, or monastic vows, that are directly or indirectly related to the original (Adi) Shankaracharya who completely reorganized the monastic system in India. Example: Swami Shivananda or Paramahamsa Yogananda

ACHARYA Teacher or spiritual guide, especially one who instructs in religious, philosophical, or spiritual disciplines.

ARKAYA The eleventh name of the sun among the 12 names or powers of the Sun.

ARTHA Wealth, prosperity, or material success. One of the four goals of human life (*Purusharthas*) in Hindu philosophy.

ASURA Demons in human-like form. Also sometimes called Daityas, they are the sworn enemies of the celestials or Devas.

ATMAN The divine flame burning in the Hrit Padma, that goes by many names including Soul, Higher Self, Divine Self. It is activated by chanting the mantra "Aham Prema."

AVATAR A divine being with no karma whatsoever who comes to Earth to perform specific beneficial tasks for humanity.

AYURVEDA Science of Life. Traditional system of medicine and holistic wellness originating in ancient India.

BHAKTI YOGA The Yoga of Devotion to God. Highest states are Prema, Divine Love, and Prapatti, total surrender and faith in God's benevolent activity.

BIJA MANTRA A seed sound that contains spiritual power that must be grown or unwrapped through its repetition, frequently as part of a longer mantra.

BRAHMA Personified Vedic God representative of the known universe and all its contents. Also called the creator of the universe in ancient story-based scriptures called the Puranas.

BRAHMANAS Scriptures which preceded the Upanishads which are said to be summaries of previous scriptures.

BUDDHA Prince Gautama, the ninth Avatar of Vishunu. Also a state of consciousness.

BUDDHI The mind in a transformed state, sometimes referred to as an enlightened state. One of the two wives of Ganesha.

BUDHA One of the many names for the planet Mercury in Vedic Astrology.

CHAKRA Literally "wheel of light" in Sanskrit. It's common meaning refers to various spiritual centers located in the subtle body. The main chakras are the six located along the spine and the seventh at the top of the head are most commonly discussed. The first or root chakra is called, "Muladhara," second chakra located at naval center is the "Svadisthana," third chakra located at Solar Plexus center is called the "Manipura," fourth chakra or heart center is the "Anahata," fifth chakra at the throat center is the "Vishuda," sixth chakra at the third eye or brow center is called the "Ajna," and the seventh chakra at the crown or top of the head is called the "Sahasrara." Also, there are dozens of other chakras in the subtle body, such as in the hands and feet.

CHAHMUNDI Form of Durga that is the most powerful in defeating seemingly unconquerable evil. She emerged from a fire ceremony conducted by 30 of the most powerful celestials. Vanquishing the evil of that time, she promised to return and defeat evil whenever her praises are sung, and her mantras are chanted.

CHANDRA The Moon in Vedic Astrology. One of the nine Navagrahas.

CLAIRAUDIENCE One of the four "Clairs." The psychic ability of subtle hearing. One may obtain information about the past, present, and future with this ability.

CLAIRVOYANCE One of the four "Clairs." The psychic ability of subtle seeing. In a similar way to Clairaudience, one may obtain information about the past, present, and future with this ability.

CLAIRSENTIENCE One of the four "Clairs." It is a form of extrasensory perception in which a person receives intuitive information through feeling or sensing energy beyond the normal five senses.

CLAIRCOGNITION One of the four "Clairs." It is the intuitive ability of "clear knowing." It refers to receiving sudden insights, ideas, or knowledge without relying on logical reasoning, prior experience, or sensory input.

COSMIC CONSCIOUSNESS Term for a state of consciousness, also called self-realization, where the essential unity of the universe is both perceived and understood.

DEVA LINGUA Divine language, referring to Sanskrit. This language is often referred to in Eastern literature as "the language of the gods."

DEVI Goddess, Feminine celestial spirit.

DEVI BHAGAVATAM (also called **DEVI BHAGAVATA PURANA**) A major Hindu scripture that focuses on the Divine Goddess (Devi) as the supreme reality.

DHANVANTARI (sometimes spelled **DHANVANTRE**) The celestial healer who appeared at the churning of the ocean of consciousness with Lakshmi. He distributed the Nectar of Immortality, giving discourse on the healing properties of plants, gems and other remedies. He is the patron saint (celestial) of Ayurveda.

DHARMA Divine law. It also refers to the proper progression of events and persons according to divine order. Means life purpose or path in life that aligns with truth, integrity, and the greater good in the Purushartas (aims of life) in Hindu Philosophy.

DIKSHA A formal initiation or sacred transmission from a guru to a disciple.

DUM Seed sound for Durga, the feminine power of protection.

EIM Seed Sound for Saraswati, the personified feminine power of knowledge, music, and sacred sound.

GANA A manifestation of collective power or divine energy, sometimes individualized and named. Also signifies a group or gathering of beings or forces.

GANAPATI or **GANESHA** The personified power of unity that removes obstacles and assigns order to various spiritual powers and abilities.

GLAUM An additional seed sound for Ganesha that works powerfully in the removal of obstacles and the energy of the earth element.

GUM Seed sound for Ganesha, the remover of obstacles.

GURU Literally, "that which dispels darkness." In this case, it is the darkness of ignorance. An enlightened spiritual teacher with the ability to transmit spiritual energy by one or more methods. Also, the name of the planet, Jupiter, in Vedic Astrology.

HANUMAN Monkey chieftain who became the foremost servant of the Avatar Rama.

HATHA YOGA The branch of Yoga that practices physical movements and postures designed to prepare the body to receive kundalini energy as it moves up the spine.

HAUM The seed sound for Shiva, the personification of universal consciousness.

HRIM The seed sound for the Hrit Padma, or Sacred Heart.

HRIT PADMA An esoteric chakra located just below the heart center, often called the Sacred Heart.

HUM Seed sound for the Vishuddha chakra located at the throat center of the subtle body.

IDA One of the main *nadis* that runs through the left side of the body, also known as the lunar energy channel in yogic anatomy. It originates in an egg-shaped bulb in the pelvic region, travels up the spine and ends in the head. Ida connects to the left nostril, and can be activated by *pranayama* (yogic breath practices), asana, and chanting Sanskrit mantras.

ISHTA DEVATA One's chosen deity. There can be a personal Ishta Devata as well as a family Ishta Devata.

JAGAD GURU An enlightened world teacher.

JAPA The repetition of mantras in an ongoing discipline or lifestyle. Japa can be audibly vocal, whispered, or completely silent. Sometimes japa can occur spontaneously, without any conscious effort. This is referred to as Ajapa japa.

JAYA Victory.

JNANA Spiritual knowledge.

JYOTISH Science of Light. Another name for the Vedic science of astrology that reveals life patterns and karmic influences.

JYOTISHA See Vedic Astrologer

KALI The most unbridled and raw form of personified feminine power in Hinduism.

KARMA The Law of Cause and Effect. The sum total of actions and thoughts that cause a reaction or return of like energy to the source that generated it. Reincarnation or rebirth continues until all karma is balanced or neutralized.

KARMA YOGA The Yoga of Action. The path of selfless action, where one performs duties and deeds without attachment to the results, offering the fruits of action to the Divine. Thus detachment is developed in the midst of daily activities.

KLIM Seed sound for attraction.

KRIM Seed sound for Kali, the feminine energy of destruction of the negative ego.

KRIYA SHAKTI The power of manifestation. The very creation of the universe is said to be a manifestation of Kriya Shakti, personified by Goddess Lakshmi.

KRIYA YOGA Form of yoga employing certain *pranayama* (breathwork), mantra, and meditation practices. It was popularized in the West by Paramahansa Yogananda.

KRISHNA Eighth Avatar of Vishnu, the preserver in the Hindu trinity (*Trimurti*). He is also worshiped as the Supreme Being by many traditions, especially within Vaishnavism. Born more than 5,000 years ago, Krishna is said to be the most complete incarnation of divinity to come to Earth. He is one of the most widely revered and beloved deities in Hinduism.

KUBERA The Hindu god of wealth, treasures, and prosperity, as well as the guardian of the North direction. Referred to as the "celestial treasurer," who works with Lakshmi, Goddess of Abundance, to distribute prosperity to those on Earth.

KUNDALINI The coiled serpentine feminine energy laying in repose at the base of the human spine. Although powering all activities in the physical and subtle bodies, it is still characterized as latent or being asleep in most people. When it awakens, new spiritual abilities manifest in individuals. Eventually it moves as an energy force up the spine in the subtle body until it reaches the crown chakra at the top of the head. At each chakra located along the spine, it releases energy leading to increased spiritual knowledge and abilities. Once the energy has reached the top of the head, the *Shakti*, another name for kundalini, meaning Divine Feminine energy, merges with Shiva (Divine Masculine energy) at the crown center. When the energy reaches the top of the head, the person can become "liberated" or a *Shiva*, free from the cycle of rebirth. Although one may choose rebirth for the purpose of service to mankind, also called a "Boddhisatva Vow." All forms of shakti are generated here including *Kriya, Jnana, Iccha, Para*, and Mantra Shakti.

KUNDALINI SHAKTI The aspect of Shakti that harmonizes an individual's birth circumstances with their karma. Electricity (both spiritual and mundane) and magnetism are manifestations of this power.

KUNDALINI YOGA A spiritual and physical practice aimed at awakening the dormant spiritual energy (kundalini) at the base of the spine and guiding it upwards through the chakras to achieve higher consciousness. This practice includes breath control (*pranayama*), meditation, postures (*asanas*), and *mudras* to awaken and elevate the energy.

LAKSHMI Goddess of Abundance and Prosperity. The creative power of Narayana, Spouse of Vishnu, and also the *shakti* of Shiva according to the Maha Lakshmi Astakam.

LAKSHMI TANTRA A text in which Lakshmi explains her

relationship with Narayana and gives teachings about the nature of the universe and its creation. She teaches in great depth and provides mantras for working with her energy.

LAM Seed sound for the first chakra (muladhara) located at the base of the spine.

LILA Drama. The divine play that represents the drama of our evolution and life, where one may rise to great heights, only to fall back many levels due to a fault or flaw.

LOTUS A type of flower that grows in the muck and mud. The Lotus is used as symbolically as reflecting the lotus of spiritual progress, which can rise from the muck of even the heaviest karma. It is often invoked as a reference to the lotus of the heart, or the heart chakra.

MAHA Great. Also a spiritual plane (*Maha Loka*) in the non-physical universe where sages and saints of high attainment are said to dwell.

MAHA MRITYUNJAYA MANTRA The great mantra to defeat death and disease. Markandeya is the Seer of this mantra, although Brahmarishi Vasistha has also been mentioned in some scriptures as the Seer.

MAHA SAMADHI Samadhi means divine absorption or embrace. Maha means great. The Great Divine Absorption is death on the physical plane. Thus, this term means leaving the physical permanently in any given incarnation.

MALA Hindu Rosary

MANDALA A divine design.

MANIPURA CHAKRA The third chakra located at the solar plexus.

MANTRA A spiritual formula producing a specific result, previously tested and verified by an ancient sage. There are millions of mantras in the oral and written records.

MANTRA SHAKTI The spiritual power or energy inherent in a mantra, activated through correct repetition, devotion, and alignment with its vibration. It is the force that awakens when sound, intention, and consciousness unite, allowing the mantra to transform the mind, purify karma, and invoke divine presence.

MANTRA SIDDHI The power one attains when one has unwrapped the power of the mantra through repetition. Mantra Siddhi is generally recognized as beginning at 125,000 repetitions of a mantra, and increases as more repetitions are completed.

MARKANDEYA A 16 year old sage who was liberated from the necessity of rebirth by a cry to Shiva. This cry subsequently became known as the Maha Mritunjaya Mantra.

MAYA Illusion or that which is not as it appears. Refers to the illusory nature of the material world, which can distract or veil the true, eternal Self.

MOKSHA Liberation or spiritual freedom. It is the ultimate goal of human life in Hindu, Jain, and Buddhist philosophies. It represents freedom from the cycle of birth, death, and rebirth (*samsara*).

MULADHARA CHAKRA The first chakra located at the base of the spine.

NADA BRAHMA The sound of the Universe.

NADIS Astral nerve tubes, similar to veins, that run through the subtle body. There are 72,000 *nadis* in the human body, which cannot be seen by any medical scan, similar to meridians in Chinese Medicine. *Nadis* connect at chakras, making them power centers because of the convergence of these subtle energy pathways. The main *nadi* is the Sushumna which is the spinal channel. There are two distribution channels on either side of the Sushumna – the *ida* on the left and *pingala* on the right side of the body.

NAMAHA "Salutations," or "I salute." There are several words for this principle. This term has a neutral ending. See also "Swaha."

NAVAGRAHAS The nine celestial bodies (or planets) in Vedic astrology believed to influence human life and destiny. *Nava* means nine, and *graha* means planet, or literally, or "to grasp." The Navagrahas include: Sun (Surya), Moon (Chandra), Mars (Mangala), Mercury (Budha), Jupiter (Guru), Venus (Shukra), Saturn (Shani), Rahu (lunar north node) and Ketu (lunar south node).

NARAYANA Personification of the source of all of this reality, including the creation of Brahma, the Creator. Also refers to the three-fold flame burning in the Hrit Padma. This apparent duality is meant to show that while we may feel apart, we are never truly separated from God or the Divine.

OM Seed sound for the sixth chakra located at the brow center in the subtle body. It is also the sound that is heard when the masculine and feminine currents, *ida* and *pingala*, meet and merge at the brow center.

PADMA Lotus in Sanskrit. Also a name that refers to Lakshmi.

PARA Supreme. Also silent or unmanifest speech. This is the silent speech perceived within deep stillness. Sages communicate through it, and adepts are heard by their teachers and masters. Ultimately, it is the most powerful form of speech. Yet, because of the background chatter of the lower mind, this divine speech can sometimes be mistaken for its imitations. Only advanced spiritual discrimination can discern the true from the false.

PARAMAHANSA The supreme swan. The swan here is another name for the Self in the Hrit Padma. Paramahansa is given to a person who has demonstrated very high spiritual attainment like Paramahansa Yogananda and Paramahansa Muktananda.

PARA SHAKTI Supreme Shakti. As a category of *shakti*, its domains are heat and light, both spiritual and material. Thus, the enlightened ones have invoked Para Shakti in one of its fullest spiritual manifestations while still in the body.

PARVATI Spouse of Shiva. Also known as Durga, Kali, and Chahmundi.

PINGALA *Pingala nadi* is located on the right side of the Sushumna (central channel) and is associated with the right nostril. It's considered the "solar" or "sun" channel, carrying warming, energizing *prana* (life force). *Pingala* is linked to masculine energy, heat, dynamism, and the sun. Breathing primarily through the right nostril is said to activate *Pingala*, increasing circulation, body temperature, and alertness.

PRANA A life force that exists in the subtle body. There are five divisions of this life force. *Prana* – situated in the region of the heart, this energy moves the lungs for inhalation and exhalation. *Apana* – This energy situated below the navel is associated with the elimination of spent energy and waste products from the physical body.

VYANA This energy pervades the whole body and gives rise to the sense of touch.

UDANA An energy centered in the throat that provides connection and disconnection of the mind from the body during deep sleep or engaged in advanced yogic practices. It does this by closing off the throat while leaving a chord or strand attached to the traveling subtle body.

SAMANA This energy at the navel center digests food and distributes the energy derived to all parts of the body, permeating the subtle body equal in every part.

PURANAS A genre of Hindu pre-history, myth, cosmology, legends, genealogies, and teachings about *dharma*, devotion, and spiritual practices.

PUJA General Sanskrit term for ceremonial worship.

RADHA Lord Krishna's lover and eternal consort who is viewed as the embodiment of pure devotion (*bhakti*), unconditional love, and the soul's longing for union with the Divine.

RAM Seed sound for the third chakra (Manipura) located at the solar plexus.

RAMA Seventh Avatar of Vishnu. One of the most revered deities in Hinduism and the central hero of the ancient epic, the Ramayana. He is considered both a historical king and a divine incarnation, who descends to uphold *dharma* (cosmic order, righteousness) and to destroy *adharma* (unrighteousness, chaos). He was the perfect ruler, husband, sage, friend and brother.

RUDRAKSHA A berry found in Northern India, that when dried and hardened is drilled and strung to form a prayer necklace called a mala. This berry is said to be especially useful in holding energy relating to Shiva and Durga (Kali).

SADGURU A God-realized teacher beyond the realms of energy-identified existence or mind-identified existence. A being firmly established in a form of enlightened activity that appears similar to daily human life. The Sadguru has a specific job of leading souls to spiritual freedom. Sadgurus have no karma in the normal sense of the word. Any seeming karma, called "Yoga Samsaras" is created by Sadgurus to hide their true nature and their work.

SADHANA Any regularly practiced spiritual discipline, such as meditation, mantra japa, or yogic practices.

SAMADHI Union with the Divine. The mind is merged, absorbed in the Divine.

SAMSARA The "ocean of rebirth" which the soul must traverse until it reaches the shores of liberation from such rebirth.

SANKALPA Intention, resolve, or heartfelt vow.

SANSKRIT Ancient language sometimes called Deva Lingua, or language of the gods. Also referred to as the Mother of Tongues since so many modern languages are derived from it.

SARASWATI She is the Hindu goddess of wisdom, knowledge, learning, speech, music, and the arts. She is one of the most revered deities in the Vedic and Hindu tradition and represents the refined, intellectual, and creative aspects of consciousness.

SATSANG Coming together with a teacher, guru, or spiritual community to hear, discuss, and reflect on spiritual teachings, such as yogic texts, or to chant mantras, sing *bhajans* (devotional songs), or meditate together.

SATURN RETURN Astrological transit when the planet Saturn (known as the lord of karma) returns to the exact point it occupied at the moment of birth. Considered a time of testing or initiation in Astrology, and marks the end of one cycle and the beginning of the next in the person's life. The first Saturn return occurs between 28-30 years old, when one is considered to become an adult astrologically. The second Saturn Return occurs between 58-60 years old when one can become a spiritual elder.

SEER A sage who has discovered a mantra or spiritual concept not previously known.

SHAKTI Power or personification of power. Another name for kundalini. The feminine potency lying dormant and latent at the base of the spine in most humans. When it becomes active, or *shakti* is awakened, individuals can develop special gifts such as the power to heal and to see into the future. In Vedic teachings, the Goddesses, Lakshmi, Parvati, Durga, Kali and Saraswati, are all expressions of the Great feminine power known as Shakti.

SHIVA Personification of consciousness in a male form. Principal deity of Hinduism, the Supreme being in Shaivism. He embodies paradox as he is both a destroyer and creator, ascetic yogi and cosmic dancer, fierce lord and compassionate benefactor.

SHRIM Seed sound for Lakshmi, the feminine energy of abundance.

SIDDHA One who has attained *siddhis*. One who is on a path of perfection of the Divine Vehicle, the physical and subtle body.

SIDDHI A seemingly magical spiritual ability or gift, such as clairvoyance or instant knowing. Plural is *siddhis*.

SUBRAMANYA Son of Shiva and Parvati, brother of Ganesha. Also known as Kartikeya, Skanda, or Murugan, is a revered Hindu deity, especially worshiped in South India. Subramanya is the youthful god of war, wisdom, and spiritual victory.

SUBTLE BODY An energy body which interpenetrates and interacts with the physical body. It is here that the chakras are located.

SWADISHTHANA CHAKRA The second chakra located at the genital center.

SWAHA Another term for "I salute" or "I offer." This term has a feminine ending. See also "Namaha."

SWAMI Hindu monk.

TANTRA A spiritual tradition from India that integrates ritual, mantra, meditation, and sacred practices to expand consciousness and unite the individual with the Divine. Rooted in both Hindu and Buddhist lineages, Tantra views the body, senses, and worldly experience as pathways to spiritual realization, rather than obstacles. Its core aim is liberation (*moksha*) and awakening through the harnessing of energy (*shakti*).

UPANISHADS A series of scriptures which are all that remain of a much larger, older body of scriptures. Originally written on palm leaves many centuries ago.

VACH Spiritual speech. An ancient name for Saraswati.

VAM Seed sound for the second chakra located at the genital center.

VEDAS The world's oldest sacred scriptures originating in India, composed in Sanskrit, and considered the foundation of Hindu philosophy, spirituality, and ritual. They consist of four main collections – Rig Veda, Yajur Veda, Sama Veda, and Atharva Veda – which contain hymns, chants, prayers, and instructions for rituals. The word Veda means "knowledge" or "wisdom," and these texts are regarded as śruti (divinely revealed knowledge) that guide both spiritual understanding and daily life.

VEDIC Pertaining to the Vedas.

VEDIC ASTROLOGER A Vedic Astrologer is a practitioner of Jyotish who interprets the positions of planets and stars to guide life, karma, and spiritual growth.

VIDYA Specific knowledge in a definitive category often denoted by another word preceding Vidya. Often contrasted with Avidya (ignorance or false knowledge). It can also denote specific fields of learning, sciences, or sacred wisdom traditions. For example: Jyotisha Vidya – the science of astrology or Sangeeta Vidya – the knowledge of music.

VINA (also spelled **VEENA**) A classical Indian stringed music instrument used in traditional Hindu music and spiritual practices. Goddess Saraswati is often depicted holding one.

VISHUDDHA CHAKRA The fifth chakra located at the throat center.

VISHNU The Vedic god of preservation. One of the principal deities of Hinduism, known as the Preserver and Protector of the universe. He maintains cosmic order (*dharma*) and often incarnates on Earth in various forms (*avatars*), such as Rama and Krishna, to restore balance and guide humanity

WORLD DHARMA The universal principles of duty, righteousness, and ethical living that sustain harmony in the world. Living in alignment with universal laws, compassion, and justice, contributing to the welfare of all beings.

YAGNA Sacrifice, usually in the sense of a ritual fire worship ceremony in which negative karma can be consumed or transmuted.

YOGA SUTRAS OF PATANJALI Foundational text of classical yoga philosophy, written by the sage Patanjali around 2,000 years ago. It consists of 196 concise sutras outlining the theory and practice of yoga. The text describes the eightfold path of Ashtanga Yoga, which includes ethical principles, discipline, posture, breath control, sense withdrawal, concentration, mediation and samadhi (union with the Divine).

bibliography

Ashley-Farrand, Thomas. *The Healing Mantras*. New York: Ballantine Wellspring Books, 1999.

Ashley-Farrand, Thomas. *The Ancient Science of Sanskrit Mantra and Ceremony*. volume 1, volume 2. Privately published 1995-96.

Ashley-Farrand, Thomas. *Teacher of Mantra Instructor Manual*. Saraswati Publications LLC, 2006.

Ashley-Farrand, Thomas. *True Stories of Spiritual Power*. Privately published 1995.

Ashley-Farrand, Thomas. *Chakra Mantras*. San Francisco: Red Wheel/Weiser Books, 2006.

Ashley-Farrand, Thomas. *Shakti Mantras*. New York: Random House Publishing, 2009.

Ashley-Farrand, Thomas. *Mantra Meditation: Change your Karma with the Power of Sacred Sound*. Lafayette: CO: Sounds True, 2013.

Bailey, Allice. *The Soul and Its Mechanism*. New York: Lucis Publishing, 1930.

Blofeld, John. Mantras. *Sacred Words of Power*. New York: E.P. Dutton, 1977.

Feuerstein, Georg. *Tantra-The Path of Ecstasy*. Boston and London: Shambala, 1998.

Frawley, David. *Tantric Yoga and the Wisdom Goddesses*. Salt Lake City: Passage Press, 1994.

Frawley, David. *Inner Tantric Yoga*. Twin Lakes, Wisconsin: Lotus Press, 2008.

Gawain, Shakti. *Creative Visualization*. New York: Bantam Books, 1983.

Gupta, Sanjukta. *Lakshmi Tantra*. Leiden, Netherlands. Brill 1972.

Hawley, Jack. *The Bhagavad Gita: A Walkthrough for Westerners*. New World Library, 2001

Keshavadas, Sadguru Sant. *Lord Ganesha*. Oakland, CA: Vishwa Dharma Publications, 1988.

Keshavadas, Sadguru Sant. *Sadguru Dattatreya*. Oakland, CA: Vishwa Dharma Publications, 1988.

Keshavadas, Sadguru Sant. *Liberation from Karma and Rebirth*. Oakland, CA: Temple of Cosmic Religion, 1970.

Keshavadas, Sadguru Sant. *Sadguru Speaks*. Oakland, CA: Temple of Cosmic Religion, 1975.

Keshavadas, Sadguru Sant. *Ramayana At A Glance*. Oakland, CA: Temple of Cosmic Religion, 1976.

Keshavadas, Sadguru Sant. *Self-Realization*. Oakland, CA: Temple of Cosmic Religion, 1976.

Keshavadas, Sadguru Sant. *Cosmic Shakti Kundalini*. Oakland, CA: Temple of Cosmic Religion, 1976.

Keshavadas, Sadguru Sant. *Life and Teachings of Sadguru Sant Keshavadas*. Oakland, CA: Temple of Cosmic Religion, 1976.

Keshavadas, Sadguru Sant. *Gayatri: The Highest Meditation*. New York: Vantage Press, 1978.

Keshavadas, Sadguru Sant. *The Purpose of Life*. New York: Vantage Press, 1978.

Keshavadas, Sadguru Sant. *Healing Techniques of the Holy East*. Oakland, CA: Vishwa Dharma Publications, 1980.

Kumar, Ravindra. *Kundalini for Beginners*. St. Paul, MN: Llewellyn Publications, 2000.

Kumar, Ravindra and Kumar Larsen, Jyttte. *The Kundalini Book of Living and Dying*. Boston: Weiser Books, 2004.

Mookerjee, Ajit. *Kundalini: The Arousal of the Inner Energy*. Rochester, VT: Destiny Books, 1986.

Radha, Swami Sivananda. *Kundalini Yoga for the West*. Spokane, WA: Timeless Books, 2011

Sutton, Komilla. *The Essentials of Vedic Astrology*. Wessex Astrologer, 1999.

Sutton, Komilla. *Indian Astrology: How to Discover the Secrets of Your Vedic Star Sign*. London: Collins & Brown Limited, 2000.

Yogananda, Paramahamsa. *Autobiography of a Yogi*. Los Angeles: Self Realization Fellowship, 1946, 1978, 1998.

Resources

Books by Sadguru Sant Keshavadas

Available through the **Temple of Cosmic Religion** at:

www.templeofcosmicreligion.org/Store/Books/books.html

Mantra Teacher Training

Gretchen Raji Carmel:

www.mantrateachertrainings.com

Mantra Workshops

Yogacharya Bharata Bill Francis Barry:

www.mantravijaya.com

Remedy Resources

Quality Malas: malaology.com/malas

Manifest Malas: Handmade Malas with Mantra japa blessings by Katherine Bennett

email: katieallenbenn@gmail.com

Beautiful Malas and Jewelry: Sky's the Limit Art

jaxxaamillion@gmail.com

Vedic Gemstones: Jack Hauck

healingems.com

Kirtan Resources

Larisa Stow and Shakti Tribe Kirtan: larisastow.com

Adam Bauer- Sacred Music and Chanting: iamadambauer.com

Deva Premal & Miten: devapremalmiten.com

Krishna Das: krishnadas.com

Jai Utall: www.jaiuttal.com

Donna De Lory: www.donnadelory.com

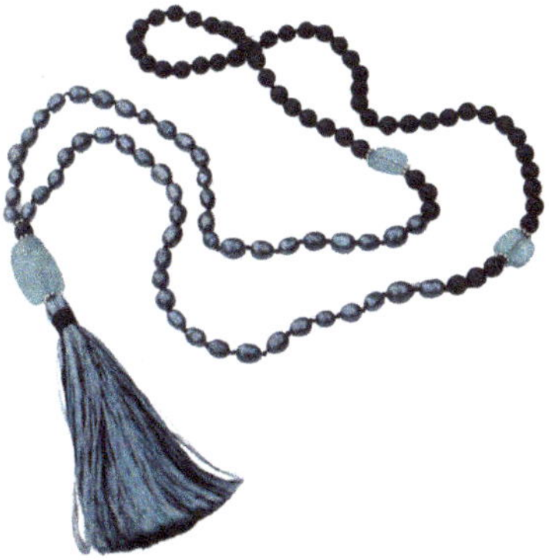

invite jill

If you would like to host a mantra workshop or event at your yoga center, other venue, or online,

OR to host *Jill as a guest on your podcast*, please email **jill@jilljardineastrology.com**

about the authors

Jill Jardine, M.A. Counseling/ Psychology, is a lifelong Astrologer and Psychic who began studying metaphysics and astrology at age 15. Since 1991, she has worked as a professional consulting astrologer and therapist. Her prior work experience was at WBUR-NPR, CBS Radio Boston, and Harvard University. Certified in Hypnotherapy and Acupressure/Shiatsu, Jill has been a Yoga teacher since 1989, as well as a Sanskrit Mantra instructor, Reverend, and Kundalini Yoga teacher. She has studied with esteemed Gurus from India and other spiritual teachers, cultivating deep insight into the mind, body, and spirit. Once told by a Vedic Jyotisha that "God and the Gurus have blessed her with the Gift of Divine Intuition," Jill is honored to share her spiritual gifts and cultivated wisdom with others. She hosts the internationally acclaimed podcast Cosmic Scene with Jill Jardine and previously led a call-in radio show on WATD 95.9 FM. Since 1992, she has maintained a thriving astrological and healing practice on Boston's South Shore and teaches workshops in Yoga, Sanskrit Mantra, Sound Healing, Past Life Regression, and Astrology.

to learn more visit

https://jilljardine.com

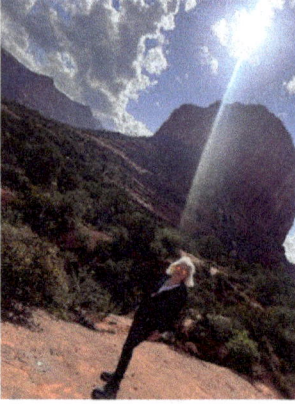

If you want to go deeper into your study on this topic, Jill offers astrology readings, mantra healing, past life regression, masterclasses, and more – guiding spiritual growth, clarity, and empowerment for life, love, and prosperity.

Astrology Readings & Guidance
Explore Western and Vedic charts for clarity on life, love, career, and major decisions. Sessions provide spiritual insight, psychic guidance, and actionable steps for positive outcomes.

Sanskrit Mantra Healing & Puja Ceremonies
Harness the power of mantras to clear obstacles, promote healing, attract prosperity, and restore emotional and spiritual balance. Puja ceremonies empower and protect on your behalf.

Past Life Regression
Recall past life memories to resolve karmic patterns, enhance self-discovery, and support spiritual growth and present-life healing.

Online Masterclasses
Learn mantra techniques to raise vibration, develop intuition, manifest prosperity, and attract love. Accessible self-study courses provide practical tools for personal and spiritual growth.

for more details and to book your sessions:

https://jilljardineastrology.com/shop

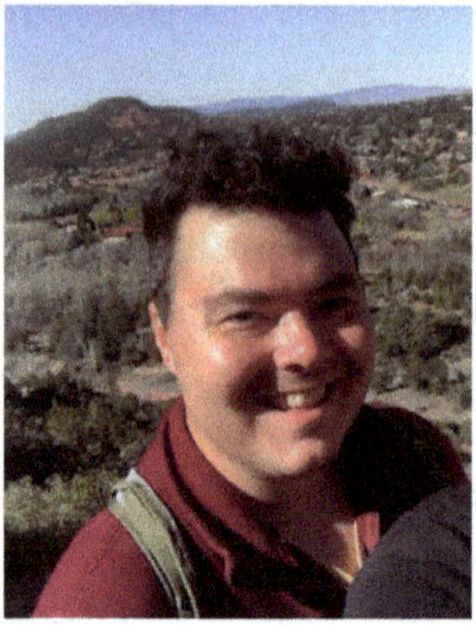

Dr. Alexi Jardine Martel is a second generation Astrologer, who specializes in Vedic Astrology, and is a certified instructor in Sanskrit Mantra. Dr. Martel is a professor of Psychology, and a Reverend in Sanskrit Mantra through Santana Dharma Satsang, the lineage of Thomas Ashley-Farrand. Alexi brings an intriguing blend of Eastern and Western perspectives to his astrology consultations. His expertise in Vedic astrology and Sanskrit mantras promises captivating insights into the mystical, and often misunderstood, world of Vedic traditions.

Dr. Martel offers various readings for those interested in diving deeper into their own Vedic chart.

- **Comprehensive Vedic Astrology Reading with Sanskrit Mantra Remedies**
  Receive an in-depth analysis of your Vedic chart, *dashas*, and transits. Alexi provides personalized Sanskrit mantra remedies to support positive outcomes and answer your questions.

- **Focused Life Planning Vedic Astrology Reading**
  Explore key life decisions and cycles – career, relationships, moves, or events. This session reveals optimal timing, astrological guidance, and actionable steps for a clearer, more positive path forward.

- **Specific Question Vedic Astrology Reading with Mantra Guidance**
  Get answers to pressing questions or life challenges. Alexi provides clarity, timing, and personalized Sanskrit mantra remedies to help you navigate transitions and take informed, confident action.

- **Sanskrit Mantra Consultation**
  Learn and receive empowered Sanskrit mantras tailored to your Vedic chart. Alexi guides mantra therapy for emotional balance, clarity, and spiritual growth.

book your sessions now at:

https://practicalsanskritmagic.com/

Cosmic Scene with Jill Jardine
PODCAST

Jill's cutting edge podcast, brings a new paradigm in the consciousness-shifting movement. Jill shares astrology updates every month, with important astrological information, and psychic hits on current and upcoming events. She interviews guests who are healers, psychics, astrologers, and leaders in the consciousness movement, and planetary awakening. Jill shares ancient sacred sound formulas that can be applied to contemporary life situations. Jill's wisdom and experience from facilitating clients to more hopeful, happier, and healthier lives will be revealed to the listeners of Cosmic Scene so they may enjoy the benefits!

Subscribe:
jilljardine.com/cosmicscene

Request to be a guest on Cosmic Scene Podcast:
jill@jilljardineastrology.com

www.ingramcontent.com/pod-product-compliance
Lightning Source LLC
Chambersburg PA
CBHW070102030426
42335CB00016B/1971

9781958150511